Nature's Answer to Viral Threats

Understanding the Potency of Plant-Based Antivirals

Liam Hawthrone

Table of Contents

INTRODUCTION

Provides an insightful examination of the efficacy of natural treatments in treating viral infections. More than ever, we need effective antiviral technologies to combat viral epidemics, which pose serious dangers to global health security. By utilizing conventional knowledge and cutting-edge scientific research, this book aims to shed light on the remarkable effectiveness of plant-based antivirals and reveal nature's undiscovered weaponry against viral infections.

Many societies have used plants' therapeutic abilities for ages and have long been valued for their medical qualities. Traditional herbal medicines have proven invaluable in treating various illnesses, including viral infections, from the Amazonian rainforests to the Asian highlands. On the strength of this rich history, modern researchers attempt to decipher the molecular workings of plant-based antivirals to get fresh perspectives on their potential as therapeutics.

This book provides readers with an in-depth overview of plant-based antivirals and their function in contemporary healthcare through a blend of historical tales, scientific findings, and clinical observations. We want to provide readers with knowledge beyond traditional methods for treating and preventing viruses by exploring essential plant components' pharmacology, effectiveness, and real-world uses. Take an insightful journey through nature's pharmacy with us as we explore the effectiveness of plant-based antivirals and imagine a time when natural medicines will be at the forefront of the battle against viral threats.

CHAPTER I

Understanding Viruses

What Are Viruses?

Viruses are peculiar organisms that exist in a state of transition between living things and non-living things. These microscopic pathogens are composed of genetic material, either DNA or RNA, covered in a capsid, a protein shell. Additionally, some viruses have an outer envelope made of lipids that are taken from the membrane of the host cell. Viruses, in contrast to bacteria, require host cells to replicate or carry out metabolic functions. Because viruses are parasitic, they are able to efficiently take over the biological machinery of their hosts and use it to manufacture more viruses.

The structure, genetic makeup, and viral transmission mechanisms exhibit extreme variation. Numerous creatures, including viruses, bacteria, plants, animals, and fungi, are susceptible to infection. Viral adaptation and evolution can occur quickly, which contributes to their ability to infect humans and other animals. Viruses are the leading cause of many diseases, including the common cold and more severe conditions such as COVID-19, HIV/AIDS, and influenza. This makes them a major global health problem.

An in-depth comprehension of the viral life cycle is needed to create successful antiviral treatments. The usual stages of a virus are assembly, release, penetration, attachment, and reproduction. Virus entry into the cell is facilitated by the attachment phase, in which specific host cell receptors are linked to viral proteins on the surface. Once within, the virus multiplies its genetic material, copies its genome, and produces viral proteins using the host cell's biological machinery. These components create newly generated virus particles, then expelled from the host cell to complete the infection cycle.

Numerous things can spread viruses, including bodily fluids, contaminated items, respiratory droplets, and vectors like ticks and mosquitoes. Viruses are difficult to treat because of their quick dissemination and capacity to modify and elude host immune responses. Vaccination, antiviral drugs, and public health strategies, including social distancing and isolation, are necessary to stop the spread of viral diseases and epidemics.

Despite their danger, viruses are vital ecological components that have influenced the evolution of life on Earth. Because they infect and regulate populations of bacteria, algae, and other microorganisms, viruses impact the dynamics of ecosystems. They can also spread genes from one species to another, increasing genetic variety and promoting evolutionary adaption. Aside from being used in gene therapy, vaccine creation, and biological process research, viruses have also been utilized in several biotechnological applications.

In brief, viruses are intricate organisms that have a significant impact on evolution, the environment, and human health. Further investigation and development are required since virology can potentially spread infectious diseases. Effective methods for diagnosing, treating, and preventing viral infections can help us reduce the impact of these hazards on the health and well-being of people worldwide. It is possible to achieve this by comprehending the principles of virology.

Viral Replication Process

Viral particles are created by the complex process of viral replication, which allows viruses to take advantage of their host's cellular machinery. To develop effective antiviral medications and combat viral infections, it is crucial to understand the intricacies of viral replication. The typical steps in the replication cycle are attachment, penetration, uncoating, replication, assembly, and release.

The virus reproduces by binding to specific receptors on its surface once it has attached itself to a host cell. This attachment is often particular because the viral proteins exclusively bind to specific types of cells or tissues. The method of attachment determines the host range and tissue tropism of the virus, affecting its ability to infect many organisms.

Once it has attached itself, the virus enters the host cell through direct membrane fusion or a process in which the host cell engulfs the virus in a vesicle tethered to its membrane. Once within the cell, the virus disassembles its capsid and uncoils, releasing its genome into the host cell's cytoplasm. Uncoating can result from various factors, including changes in the pH or the activity of the host cell's enzymes.

After the viral genome has been released into the host cell, the next stage of viral replication involves the replication of the viral genome and the synthesis of viral proteins. Replication methods for viruses vary depending on the type of virus and the composition of its genome. DNA viruses usually need host cell DNA polymerases to replicate their genomes, but RNA viruses can encode their RNA-dependent RNA polymerase or rely on host cell replication machinery. Viruses use their genome as a template to create their RNA or protein using the host cell's protein synthesis machinery.

Assembling freshly created viral proteins and genomes to create new viral particles is known as assembly.
Depending on the virus, this may occur in specific cellular compartments or throughout the cell membrane. During assembly, various components are packed and integrated

into new viral particles, including the envelope, capsid, and viral DNA.

Eventually, the newly created virus particles are released from the host cell to propagate the infection and infect additional cells. Different viruses are released in different ways. For example, encapsulated viruses may bud from the host cell membrane, while non-enclosed viruses lyse the host cell to release viral particles.

In summary, for viruses to multiply, they need to seize control of the host cell's internal components. This method involves several steps. Researchers can develop customized antiviral therapies to break the replication cycle and prevent viral infections by understanding the mechanics underpinning viral replication. Furthermore, knowledge of viral replication can guide the development of vaccinations and other interventions to prevent viral infections and maintain public health.

Common Viral Threats to Human Health

Viruses are common infectious organisms that, wherever they exist, represent a severe risk to human health. Everyone is susceptible to viral illnesses, which range from the common cold to more severe infections, including influenza, COVID-19, and HIV/AIDS. These illnesses may cause morbidity, mortality, and financial hardship. Creating preventative, diagnostic, and therapeutic plans requires understanding common viral threats to human health.

The common cold is one of the most frequent viral infections that affect humans, and adenoviruses, coronaviruses, and rhinoviruses mainly cause it. Common colds are generally harmless and self-limiting, but they can occasionally be uncomfortable and inconvenient, especially for older people, small children, and people with compromised immune systems. More accurately, respiratory droplets from sick people disseminate the virus that causes most cases of the common cold. Rhinoviruses are incredibly contagious.

Another common viral respiratory infection that affects millions of individuals annually worldwide is influenza, commonly known as the flu. The three primary influenza virus types, A, B, and C are members of the Orthomyxoviridae family. The most vicious influenza viruses are those that generate seasonal epidemics and sporadic pandemics, which have the potential to cause high rates of hospitalization and mortality. Flu symptoms include fever, coughing, sore throats, body aches, and fatigue. Severe cases can lead to sinus infections, pneumonia, and respiratory problems.

To weaken the immune system and lessen the body's capacity to fend off infection, the HIV retrovirus targets explicitly CD4+ T cells. Acquired immunodeficiency syndrome (AIDS), which is typified by a compromised immune system and heightened vulnerability to opportunistic infections and certain malignancies, can arise from HIV infection. Antiretroviral therapy (ART) advancements notwithstanding, HIV/AIDS continues to be a primary worldwide health concern, especially in low-resource countries such as sub-Saharan Africa.

Another well-known virus that is dangerous to human health is the hepatitis B virus (HBV), which primarily affects the liver and can cause cirrhosis, hepatocellular carcinoma, and acute and chronic hepatitis. The transmission of contaminated blood or body fluids from mother to child, sharing of needles, and sexual contact are all possible routes of infection. An estimated 257 million people worldwide suffer from a chronic HBV infection, making it the primary cause of liver-related illness and mortality.

There has been a lot of discussion about the possibility that freshly identified coronaviruses could cause worldwide outbreaks and central respiratory diseases. Coughing, fever, and difficulty breathing of breath are the hallmarks of the severe acute respiratory syndrome (SARS) epidemic, which is caused by the severe acute respiratory syndrome coronavirus (SARS-CoV), which first appeared in 2002–2003. 2012 saw the emergence of the Middle East respiratory syndrome coronavirus or MERS-CoV. Middle East respiratory syndrome (MERS), whose symptoms can range from moderate respiratory illness to severe pneumonia and organ failure, was brought on by it.

The coronavirus disease 2019 (COVID-19) pandemic, associated with the new SARS-CoV-2 virus, is the most recent and potentially significant viral threat to human health. After being discovered in Wuhan, China, in December 2019, COVID-19 swiftly spread over the world, killing and infecting millions of people. Some symptoms, including fever, coughing, dyspnea, exhaustion, loss of taste or smell, and digestive problems, are associated with COVID-19. Severe episodes, particularly in older adults and those with underlying medical issues, can develop into multiorgan failure and acute respiratory distress syndrome (ARDS).

The COVID-19 epidemic has not only harmed people's health but also severely affected daily life, economy, and healthcare systems. The quick spread of SARS-CoV-2 emphasizes how interconnected the globe is today and how crucial international collaboration is in the battle against newly emerging infectious diseases. Efforts to stop the COVID-19 virus have mainly focused on public health initiatives such as mask wear, social distancing, hand cleanliness, testing, contact tracing, and vaccines.

Due to their ability to spread to a broad spectrum of infectious diseases, viruses provide a varied and persistent risk to human health. From the common cold to newly developing pandemics like COVID-19, viruses continue to elude our comprehension of the mechanics behind infectious diseases and our capacity to create effective therapeutic interventions. By allowing us to anticipate and reduce potential viral dangers, investments in research, surveillance, and public health infrastructure can safeguard the health and welfare of communities everywhere.

CHAPTER II

The Rise of Antiviral Resistance

Challenges with Traditional Antiviral Drugs

Traditional antiviral medications have been a vital part of treating viral infections for many years because they provide symptomatic relief, inhibit viral reproduction, and stop viruses from spreading throughout the body. However, standard antiviral medications need some help with their usefulness in fully addressing viral threats despite their widespread usage and efficacy against certain viral diseases. Things like reduced effectiveness, side effects, viral resistance, and the limited range of action of many antiviral medications cause these difficulties.

The formation of viral resistance, which occurs when viruses acquire changes that make them less vulnerable to the effects of antiviral treatments, is one of the main problems with conventional antiviral drugs. This behavior is ubiquitous when it comes to viruses based on RNA, such as the human immunodeficiency virus (HIV) and influenza virus, because of the high rates of mutation linked to RNA replication. Several factors, such as changes in drug metabolic pathways, mutations in viral target proteins, and selection pressure from insufficient treatment dosage or adherence, can result in viral resistance. The long-term effectiveness of antiviral medication is severely hampered by the emergence of viral resistance, which calls for creating innovative therapeutic approaches to get around this problem.

The poor effectiveness of standard antiviral medications against some viral pathogens—particularly those with intricate reproduction cycles or innate resistance mechanisms—presents another difficulty. Hepatitis C virus (HCV), for instance, is difficult to eradicate with traditional antiviral medications due to its propensity for prolonged infection and fast mutation. Herpesviruses, including cytomegalovirus (CMV) and herpes simplex virus (HSV), can infect host cells and cause latent infections that last a lifetime, making them resistant to conventional antiviral treatment. The management of chronic viral infections is complicated by the inability to complete viral clearance or prevent viral reactivation, which calls for creating new therapeutic modalities.

Another major obstacle to the clinical usage of conventional antiviral medications is their adverse effects. Many antiviral drugs have side effects that can range from minor gastrointestinal distress to severe organ damage, making it difficult for patients to tolerate and comply with them. For instance, lactic acidosis, mitochondrial toxicity, and bone marrow suppression are linked to nucleoside analogs, which are prescribed to treat HIV and hepatitis B virus (HBV) infections. Analogously, gastrointestinal symptoms, neuropsychiatric side effects, and allergic responses can result from neuraminidase inhibitors prescribed to treat influenza virus infections. Traditional antiviral medications have a risk-benefit profile that must be carefully considered to decrease the possibility of side effects and improve patient results.

Furthermore, conventional antiviral medications frequently have a narrow spectrum of activity, which means that only a small subset of viral infections or strains may be effectively treated with them. For instance, neuraminidase inhibitors, such as oseltamivir, primarily work against influenza A and B viruses. Still, their effectiveness against other respiratory viruses, including rhinovirus or respiratory syncytial virus (RSV), may be restricted. Analogous nucleosides, such as acyclovir, are exclusive to herpesviruses and might not work against unrelated viral families. The absence of antiviral drugs with a broad range of activity hinders attempts to counter new viral threats. It creates innovative antiviral tactics with more extensive activity profiles.

In summary, several obstacles prevent conventional antiviral medications from effectively addressing viral threats broadly. Some of these issues include a narrow spectrum of action, side effects, limited efficiency against specific viral infections, and the emergence of viral resistance. To overcome these obstacles, antiviral medication development will need to continue researching and innovating, emphasizing finding new therapeutic targets, improving drug delivery methods, and deepening our knowledge of viral pathogenesis. By overcoming these obstacles, we can create drugs for antiviral purposes that are safer and more effective in the fight against viral infections, thus enhancing public health outcomes.

Need for Alternative Solutions

Alternative approaches to treating viral infections are desperately needed, as seen by the rise of viral threats and the problems with conventional antiviral medications. Traditional antiviral medications have been essential in treating viral illnesses. Still, they have drawbacks such as limited effectiveness, side effects, and a limited range of activity. These difficulties underline how crucial it is to investigate alternate viral prevention, diagnosis, and therapy methods, such as creating brand-new antiviral drugs, immunotherapies, and home cures.

Creating novel antiviral medicines with distinct modes of action and broader activity profiles offers a viable solution to the drawbacks of conventional antiviral medications. This involves investigating novel drug targets, such as host-virus interactions, viral entry and fusion, or viral proteins implicated in critical cellular functions.

Researchers can create antiviral medications that are more effective against a broader variety of viral pathogens and less prone to resistance by focusing on unique viral vulnerabilities. Improvements in drug discovery tools, including computational modeling, high- throughput screening, and structure-based drug design, have made finding and optimizing new antiviral agents with improved potency and selectivity easier.

Using immunotherapies, which combine traditional small-molecule medications with the immune system's ability to identify and eradicate viral viruses, a promising strategy for treating viral infections is being explored. The creation of therapeutic vaccinations, adoptive cell treatments, and monoclonal antibodies that target immunological checkpoints or viral antigens implicated in antiviral immunity are examples of this. Specifically, monoclonal antibodies have demonstrated potential as antiviral treatments against respiratory syncytial virus (RSV), influenza virus, and SARS-CoV-2. Immunotherapies supplement conventional antiviral medications by enhancing the immune system's response to viral pathogens, which may result in long-lasting protection against viral infections.

Another exciting option for creating substitute antiviral treatments is using natural therapies made from plants, fungi, and other natural sources. Since many plants have strong antiviral qualities, traditional herbal therapy has been utilized for ages to treat viral infections. These organic substances frequently target several stages of the viral replication cycle, which reduces their susceptibility to resistance and allows them to work in concert with traditional antiviral medications to produce synergistic effects. In addition, compared to synthetic pharmaceuticals, natural therapies tend to be well-tolerated and have fewer side effects, which makes them appealing candidates for additional research and development.

Technological developments in biotechnology, such as gene editing tools like CRISPR-Cas9, present intriguing prospects for developing novel antiviral approaches that specifically target viral genomes or host proteins crucial to viral replication. CRISPR-based methods, for instance, can be used to modify host cell components involved in viral infection, selectively edit viral genomes, or interfere with the expression of viral genes. Researchers can create highly targeted antiviral therapies with the potential to eradicate viral infections and stop viral transmission by utilizing the accuracy and adaptability of CRISPR technology.

Furthermore, the antiviral medication research and development field could be transformed by incorporating digital technologies like machine learning, artificial intelligence (AI), and big data analytics. With the aid of these technologies, scientists may examine enormous collections of clinical data, protein structures, and viral genomic sequences to find new therapeutic targets, anticipate interactions between drugs and viruses, and enhance the safety and efficacy of drug candidates. Digital technologies can also help with the quick design, synthesis, and testing of antiviral compounds, speeding up the drug development process and lowering the time and expense needed to introduce new antiviral medications to the market.

In conclusion, considering the drawbacks of conventional antiviral medications and the advent of new viral dangers, there is an unprecedented need for alternate approaches to treating viral infections. By embracing innovation and interdisciplinary collaboration, researchers can create new antiviral drugs, immunotherapies, and natural treatments that could completely change how viral illnesses are treated and prevented. These substitute approaches give hope for a future in which viral diseases are successfully managed and global health security is reinforced against new viral threats.

Introduction to Plant-Based Antivirals as a Promising Option

Investigating plant-based antivirals has become a viable strategy for treating viral infections in light of the growing risks of viruses and conventional antiviral medications' shortcomings. Many cultures have long recognized the therapeutic benefits of plants, and they have been using them for ages to treat various ailments. Plants have been used for centuries as a great source of bioactive chemicals with various pharmacological actions, including antiviral capabilities. These practices can be traced back to the indigenous remedies of the Amazon jungle and the ancient herbal traditions of Ayurveda and Traditional Chinese Medicine.

Historical documents attest to the medicinal application of numerous plant species in customary healing practices, which extends the history of using plants as natural treatments for viral infections back thousands of years. Indigenous civilizations have created complex systems of knowledge about medicinal plants, transmitting this information through written texts, empirical observations, and oral traditions. The production of decoctions, infusions, poultices, and tinctures using plant parts—such as roots, leaves, bark, and fruits—that are each thought to have particular medicinal qualities is a common practice in these traditional herbal medicines.

Modern scientific discoveries have clarified the mechanisms of action and revealed the biochemical underpinnings of many traditional plant-based medicines' antiviral activity, thereby validating their usefulness. Numerous studies have shown that plant chemicals have antiviral properties against various viral infections, such as hepatitis viruses, herpes viruses, influenza viruses, respiratory viruses, and HIV. These substances show a variety of modes of action, such as modulating the host immune system's reaction to viral infection and inhibiting viral entry, replication, transcription, translation, and assembly.

Plant-based antivirals have several benefits, one of which is their broad-spectrum activity, which allows them to combat various virus species or strains. Plant-derived chemicals have been found to have pleiotropic effects, meaning that they target many steps in the viral replication cycle and work in concert to combat viral infections. This contrasts with traditional antiviral medications, often targeting specific viral proteins or pathways. Plant-based antivirals are more effective against a broader range of viral infections and less likely to develop viral resistance by targeting several targets.

In addition, plant-based antivirals have superior safety profiles and a decreased chance of side effects compared to conventional antiviral medications. They are more readily available and reasonably priced, especially in environments with limited resources. For millennia, people have safely used various substances produced from plants as nutritional supplements or herbal treatments. The ecological impact of producing antiviral drugs can also be reduced by employing sustainable and eco-friendly methods to grow and extract medicinal plants.

Phytochemistry, pharmacology, and botanical medicine are seeing a boom in research and development because of the increasing interest in plant-based antivirals. Researchers are delving further into the enormous variety of plant species that may be found in various ecosystems across the globe, testing plant extracts and isolated chemicals for antiviral activity and figuring out the molecular processes that underlie their therapeutic benefits. Novel antiviral agents with solid action against newly developing viral diseases, such as coronaviruses, flaviviruses, and filoviruses, have been found thanks to this interdisciplinary approach.

In summary, plant-based antivirals are viable for Nature's Answer to Viral Threats since they provide a safe, healthy, and efficient substitute for conventional antiviral medications. Plant-derived chemicals possess a wealth of pharmacological diversity, favorable safety profiles, and broad-spectrum activity that could transform viral infection diagnosis, treatment, and prevention. Researchers can unleash the full therapeutic potential of plants and pave the road for a healthier, more robust future in the face of viral threats by embracing the knowledge of traditional herbal medicine and utilizing the strength of modern science.

CHAPTER III

Exploring Plant-Based Antivirals

History of Plant-Based Medicine

Evidence of herbal medicines dates back thousands of years, making the history of plant-based medicine as old as human civilization. Throughout history, plants have been essential to traditional healing methods worldwide, providing various tribes and civilizations with food, medicine, and spiritual connections. Plants have long been valued for their therapeutic qualities and excellent healing potential, from the age-old herbal traditions of Ayurveda and Traditional Chinese Medicine (TCM) to the native healing techniques of Native American tribes and the shamanic ceremonies of Amazonian civilizations.

Plant-based medicine has its roots in prehistoric times when people used intuition, observation, and trial-and-error to find plants with therapeutic qualities. Based on archeological findings, our forefathers utilized various plants, such as leaves, roots, bark, seeds, and flowers, for therapeutic purposes. Each plant kind was thought to have unique therapeutic qualities. Traditional herbal medicine has its roots in the knowledge of medicinal plants that have been passed down through the years through oral traditions, folklore, and shamanic rituals.

Ayurveda is one of the earliest documented systems of plant-based treatment, having roots over 5,000 years ago in ancient India. Translating to "the science of life," Ayurveda is a holistic medical system that strongly emphasizes maintaining a balance between the mind, body, and spirit for optimum health and well-being. Plants are categorized in Ayurvedic medicine based on their taste (rasa), energy (virya), and post-digestive effect (vipaka). Each plant is believed to have unique medicinal qualities that can help the body regain harmony and balance.

Similarly, Traditional Chinese Medicine (TCM) has over 2,000 years of documented history using botanicals for therapeutic purposes. Traditional Chinese Medicine (TCM) bases its theory of health and illness on the idea that Qi, vital energy, and the body's Yin and Yang energies are balanced. Thousands of plant species are classed based on their energy qualities and medicinal effects, and herbs are essential to traditional Chinese medicine (TCM). TCM practitioners use complicated herbal formulae that are customized for each patient, frequently blending several plants to maximize benefits and reduce adverse effects.

Indigenous societies worldwide have also created complex systems of plant-based medicine, drawing on their ecological settings, customs, and knowledge systems. For example, Native American tribes use plants that are native to North and South America and have a profound awareness of their medicinal qualities to cure a variety of conditions, such as wounds, infections, and chronic diseases. Comparably, the native populations in the Amazon rainforest possess an extensive collection of medicinal plants, many of which have antiviral solid qualities and have been used for many years to treat infectious disorders.

Plants have long been valued for their capacity to heal the body and the psyche, acting as mediums for sacramental sacraments, spiritual enlightenment, and individual development. Psychoactive plants like iboga, peyote, and ayahuasca are used in holy ceremonies by shamanic tribes all over the world to communicate with the spirit realm, produce altered states of consciousness, and aid in healing. These plant-based remedies provide significant understandings of the nature of reality, the interdependence of all life, and the mysteries of existence.

Traditional plant-based cures were replaced with synthetic medications and pharmaceutical interventions as modern medicine gained popularity in the 19th and 20th centuries. However, as individuals look for natural, holistic alternatives to traditional treatments, there has been a renaissance of interest in plant-based therapy in recent decades. The development of new bioactive chemicals with robust therapeutic characteristics and the rediscovery of many ancient herbal treatments result from advances in scientific study, pharmacology, and botanical medicine.

As more people become aware of the benefits of botanical treatments for enhancing health and wellness, researchers, medical professionals, and patients are turning to plant-based medicine in more significant numbers. Plants are now again recognized as potent partners in the fight against disease, from producing standardized herbal extracts and nutritional supplements to incorporating herbal medicine into mainstream healthcare systems. The investigation of plant-based antivirals offers a promising new direction in the search for Nature's Answer to Viral risks, given the rise of viral risks and the shortcomings of traditional antiviral medications. We can realize the full promise of plant-based medicine and provide the groundwork for a more robust, healthy human future by utilizing the vast pharmacological diversity of plants and the knowledge of conventional medical methods.

Diversity of Plant Compounds with Antiviral Properties

Nature offers an abundant supply of chemicals found in plants that have strong antiviral effects in the continuous fight against viral threats. This variety of compounds generated from plants offers a viable way to fight viral infections. Many societies have used plants for their medicinal qualities throughout history, and current scientific research still reveals these natural substances' potential for treatment. The range of antiviral chemicals obtained from plants is extensive and diverse, ranging from modern medications to conventional herbal therapies.

Polyphenols are among the most well-known classes of antiviral substances present in plants. Numerous health advantages, including antiviral activity, have been thoroughly investigated for these bioactive compounds found in abundance in fruits, vegetables, and herbs. Flavonoids, tannins, and phenolic acids are examples of polyphenols that demonstrate a variety of antiviral actions, such as modulating host immunological responses, inhibiting viral reproduction, and obstructing viral entry into host cells. Plants rich in polyphenols that have demonstrated antiviral effects include licorice (Glycyrrhiza spp.), elderberries (Sambucus spp.), and green tea (Camellia sinensis).

Terpenoids are yet another group of plant chemicals that have strong antiviral properties. These organic substances, which are present in resinous plant exudates and essential oils, have a variety of biological functions, including the ability to combat viruses. Terpenoids with antiviral qualities, such as limonene, eucalyptol, and thymol, can combat various viruses, including respiratory syncytial virus, herpes simplex virus, and influenza.

Terpenoids-rich plants, such thyme (Thymus vulgaris), eucalyptus (Eucalyptus spp.), and citrus fruits (Citrus spp.), have long been used for their antiviral qualities and are still being researched for their possible medical uses. Numerous plant species contain nitrogen-containing substances called alkaloids, which also show encouraging antiviral qualities. Examples are quinine from cinchona (Cinchona spp.), caffeine from coffee (Coffea spp.), and berberine from goldenseal (Hydrastis canadensis). These alkaloids have been demonstrated to boost host immune responses, prevent viral assembly, and decrease viral replication. Furthermore, a few alkaloids have particular antiviral properties against RNA viruses, which suggests that they could be used to create brand-new antiviral medications.

Moreover, plant-derived polysaccharides with immunomodulatory and antiviral qualities, such as mannans and beta-glucans, have drawn interest. These complex carbohydrates improve the host's capacity to fight viral infections by inducing innate and adaptive immune responses. Plants high in polysaccharides, such as medicinal mushrooms like reishi (Ganoderma spp.) and astragalus root (Astragalus membranaceus), are being studied for their potential in antiviral therapy and have been employed in traditional medicine systems for their immunomodulatory effects.

Exploring nature's pharmacopeia to pursue efficacious antiviral drugs is crucial, as evidenced by the wide range of chemicals produced by plants that possess antiviral activities. To fully realize these natural chemicals' medicinal potential, though, in-depth scientific research is needed to clarify their modes of action, maximize their effectiveness, and guarantee their safety for human consumption. Furthermore, maintaining this vital supply of antiviral medicines for future generations depends on the sustainable production and preservation of medicinal plants.

To sum up, various plant chemicals with antiviral characteristics provide a potential approach to counteracting viral risks. Numerous plant species include polyphenols, terpenoids, alkaloids, and polysaccharides that exhibit vigorous antiviral activity via various modes of action. By utilizing these natural chemicals' therapeutic potential, we can create new antiviral drugs that will lessen the impact of viral infections on people's health worldwide. Furthermore, the study of nature's pharmacy yields helpful remedies. It emphasizes how crucial biodiversity preservation is to the health of ecosystems and people alike.

Examples of Plant-Based Antiviral Remedies from Different Cultures

Many societies have used plants for their therapeutic qualities throughout human history, including treating viral diseases. Plant-based medicine has a long history that crosses continents and includes various botanicals with strong antiviral properties. Utilizing plant-based therapies to counteract viral dangers, from old herbal medicines to contemporary pharmacological research, provides an intriguing look into nature's pharmacy. By examining plant-based antiviral medicines from various cultures, we may recognize the variety of methods and the abundance of botanical knowledge inherited over the years.

Many herbs have been utilized for centuries in traditional Chinese medicine (TCM) for their antiviral qualities. Astragalus membranaceus, sometimes called milkvetch root or Huang Qi, is one prominent example. TCM regards astragalus as having excellent immune-stimulating properties and frequently prescribes it to fortify the body's resistance to viral illnesses. Studies have indicated that astragalus possesses antiviral properties in the form of polysaccharides and flavonoids, especially against respiratory viruses, including respiratory syncytial virus (RSV) and influenza. Furthermore, astragalus has been studied for its ability to modulate immunological responses and reduce inflammation, thereby mitigating the severity of viral respiratory infections.

The traditional Indian medical system known as Ayurveda has traditionally valued herbs for their medicinal qualities. One such plant frequently utilized in Ayurveda for its antiviral and immune-boosting properties is tulsi, also known as holy basil (Ocimum sanctum). Tulsi is thought to strengthen the immune system and lower inflammation, which increases the body's resistance to viral infections. Research has demonstrated that holy basil extracts have antiviral properties against various viruses, such as dengue, herpes simplex, and influenza. The antiviral qualities of tulsi essential oil are further enhanced by the presence of substances like rosmarinic acid and eugenol, also used in Ayurvedic medicine.

Plants are essential to the therapeutic techniques handed down through the centuries in the traditional medical systems of indigenous nations. For instance, a wide variety of plant species with therapeutic qualities, many of which have shown antiviral activity, may be found in the Amazon jungle. Indigenous communities have utilized the woody vine known as cat's claw (Uncaria tomentosa), native to the Amazon basin, for generations due to its antiviral and immune-boosting qualities. Studies have demonstrated that components in a cat's claw, like polyphenols and alkaloids, have antiviral properties against influenza, HIV, and herpes simplex virus.

Additionally, studies have looked into cat claw's capacity to control immunological responses and lessen inflammation, which would improve the body's defenses against viral infections.

Many plants are prized for their antiviral qualities and are used to treat various viral diseases in African traditional medicine. Sutherlandia frutescens, commonly referred to as the "cancer bush" or "balloon pea," is a native of southern Africa and is utilized historically for its antiviral and immune-stimulating properties. Research has demonstrated that Sutherlandia frutescens extracts have antiviral properties against various viruses, including the virus that causes herpes simplex (HIV). Sutherlandia is a beneficial cure in African traditional medicine because it also contains bioactive components, including flavonoids and saponins, that contribute to its antiviral capabilities.

Plants have been used for centuries in traditional European herbalism to treat various illnesses, including viral infections. Purple coneflower, or Echinacea purpurea, is a perennial herb native to North America. It has been used extensively in European herbal medicine due to its antiviral and immune-stimulating properties. Studies have demonstrated that bioactive components found in Echinacea extracts, such as polysaccharides and alkamides, have antiviral properties against respiratory viruses, such as the rhinovirus and influenza virus. Additionally, studies have looked into Echinacea's capacity to boost immune responses and lessen the intensity and length of viral respiratory infections.

To sum up, instances of plant-based antiviral treatments from many cultures demonstrate the wide range of botanical knowledge and customary medical procedures found worldwide. Plants are still seen as essential resources in the fight against viral dangers and are used in traditional Chinese medicine, Ayurveda, and environments ranging from the African savannah to the Amazon rainforest. By investigating the antiviral qualities of plants from various cultural traditions, we can learn more about nature's pharmacy and utilize botanicals' therapeutic potential for the good of humankind. Furthermore, maintaining access to these priceless treatments for future generations depends on the sustainable cultivation of medicinal plants and preserving traditional knowledge.

CHAPTER IV

Mechanisms of Action

How Plant Compounds Combat Viruses

Since viruses can cause a wide range of infectious diseases that severely hinder medical science, they are a persistent threat to human health. Plant chemicals with strong antiviral capabilities have become significant tools in the ongoing fight against viral diseases. Plants have evolved intricate biochemical defense mechanisms against viruses and other diseases during millennia of evolution. These natural defenses frequently entail the production of specific chemicals that not only shield the plant but also provide medical advantages to people. By clarifying how plant-based compounds fight viruses, scientists have discovered an abundance of promising antiviral drugs that can transform the management and avoidance of viral illnesses.

Plant chemicals interfere with the replication of viruses as one of their primary methods of fighting them. Many viruses need host cells to grow and disperse throughout the body. Plant substances can interfere with several phases of the viral replication cycle, preventing the virus's spread. For instance, it has been demonstrated that polyphenols like epigallocatechin gallate (EGCG), present in green tea, prevent the influenza virus from replicating by interfering with the production of viral RNA and protein. Similarly, terpenoids found in thyme and other aromatic plants, such as thymol, have antiviral properties that rupture the integrity of viral membranes and prevent viral entry into host cells.

Plant chemicals can improve antiviral defenses by modulating host immunological responses and targeting virus replication. The immune system is essential for identifying and getting rid of viral infections from the body. Certain substances produced from plants, such as the polysaccharides in reishi (Ganoderma spp.) and other medicinal mushrooms, have been demonstrated to activate immune cells and improve their capacity to fight viral infections. By strengthening the body's natural defenses against viruses, these immunomodulatory effects might lessen the intensity and length of infections.

Moreover, plant components have antioxidant qualities that help lessen viruses' harm. Viruses frequently cause oxidative stress in their hosts, which damages tissue and causes inflammation. Plant-based antioxidants like flavonoids and carotenoids aid in scavenging free radicals and lessening the oxidative damage brought on by viral replication. For instance, it has been demonstrated that quercetin, a flavonoid found in large amounts in fruits and vegetables, inhibits the growth of respiratory viruses such as influenza and rhinovirus, and it has anti-inflammatory and antioxidant properties.

Plant chemicals also work against viruses by preventing the attachment and penetration of viruses into host cells. Most of the time, viruses need to bind to particular receptors on the surface of their hosts to enter and start an infection. By attaching to or hiding these receptors, plant substances can inhibit viral attachment and stop viruses from attaching to and infecting host cells. One class of proteins in many plants, called lectins, can bind to viral glycoproteins, preventing the virus from attaching to host cell receptors. Furthermore, several plant substances can interfere with viral entrance machinery or envelope proteins, which stop viruses from fusing and infecting host cells.

Additionally, when combined, plant chemicals have synergistic effects that increase their antiviral efficacy against various viruses. Several plant substances with complementing antiviral qualities are frequently used in traditional herbal treatments, increasing their efficiency compared to single compounds. For instance, traditional medicine has used ginger (Zingiber officinale) and licorice root (Glycyrrhiza spp.) to treat respiratory infections. Glycyrrhizin, a substance with antiviral qualities, is present in licorice, while ginger has anti-inflammatory and immune-boosting qualities. Combined, these plant- based chemicals offer a diverse strategy for battling viral infections.

In addition, plant chemicals have the benefit of being more widely available and reasonably priced when compared to synthetic antiviral medications. Many plant-based medicines are easily accessible as dietary or herbal supplements and have been utilized for centuries in traditional medical systems worldwide. Because of its accessibility, plant-based antiviral medicines are especially beneficial in areas with limited resources where access to traditional medical treatments may be restricted. Furthermore, compared to synthetic medications, the use of plant chemicals for antiviral objectives is frequently linked to fewer adverse effects and a lower risk of developing drug resistance.

In conclusion, antiviral drugs with various modes of action and therapeutic advantages can be abundant in plant substances. Plant chemicals provide a diverse strategy to fight viral infections because of their capacity to suppress viral replication, modify immunological responses, reduce oxidative stress, or interfere with viral entry into host cells. Furthermore, they present a viable option for creating innovative antiviral treatments due to their synergistic effects, accessibility, and relative safety. Researchers and medical professionals can keep investigating the possibilities of plant compounds as nature's solution to viral dangers by utilizing the power of nature's pharmacy.

Targeting Viral Replication and Entry

While they can cause a wide range of infectious diseases with severe socioeconomic consequences, viruses pose serious hazards to human health. Targeting viral replication and entry into host cells is one of the most essential tactics in the fight against viral infections since these activities are necessary for spreading and multiplying viruses throughout the body. Viral replication and entrance pathways are disrupted by a wide range of substances found in nature, which are derived from plants, microbes, and other sources. These compounds have antiviral solid capabilities. Researchers have created innovative methods to fight viral infections and found promising targets for antiviral therapy by clarifying the molecular mechanisms behind viral entry and reproduction.

The production of viral proteins and nucleic acids within host cells is crucial in the intricate viral replication process. Many viruses replicate their genetic material and create viral progeny by relying on the cellular machinery of their hosts. It has been demonstrated that substances derived from plants can obstruct several phases of viral replication, preventing the infection from spreading. For instance, it has been demonstrated that green tea's polyphenols, such as epigallocatechin gallate (EGCG), prevent the influenza virus from replicating by interfering with the production of viral RNA and protein expression.

Similarly, terpenoids found in thyme and other aromatic plants, such as thymol, have antiviral properties that rupture the integrity of viral membranes and prevent viral replication. Plant chemicals can efficiently limit viral proliferation and lessen the severity of viral infections by targeting critical enzymes involved in viral replication, such as viral polymerases and proteases.

Plant chemicals can delay the onset of infection by interfering with the entry of viruses into host cells and targeting their reproduction. Most of the time, viruses need to bind to particular receptors on the surface of their hosts to enter and start an infection. Compounds originating from plants can either bind to or mask these receptors, thus blocking the attachment of viruses and their ability to infect host cells. One class of proteins in many plants, called lectins, can bind to viral glycoproteins and prevent the virus from attaching itself to host cell receptors. Furthermore, several plant substances can interfere with viral entrance machinery or envelope proteins, which stop viruses from fusing and infecting host cells. Plant chemicals can effectively stop the propagation of viruses within the body and prevent the establishment of infection by targeting the processes via which viruses enter the body.

Moreover, plant chemicals' synergistic actions can strengthen their antiviral efficacy against various viruses. Several plant substances with complementing antiviral qualities are frequently used in traditional herbal treatments, increasing their efficiency compared to single compounds. For instance, traditional medicine has used ginger (Zingiber officinale) and licorice root (Glycyrrhiza spp.) to treat respiratory infections. Glycyrrhizin, a substance with antiviral qualities, is present in licorice, while ginger has anti-inflammatory and immune-boosting qualities. Combined, these plant chemicals offer a diverse strategy for battling viral infections. They are capable of efficiently focusing on viral entrance and reproduction pathways.

Furthermore, plant-derived chemicals have many benefits over traditional antiviral medications, such as ease of use, fewer side effects, and affordability. Many plant-based medicines are easily accessible as dietary additives or herbal supplements and have been utilized for ages in traditional medical systems worldwide. Because of its accessibility, plant-based antiviral medicines are especially beneficial in areas with limited resources where access to traditional medical treatments may be restricted. Furthermore, compared to synthetic medications, the use of plant chemicals for antiviral objectives is frequently linked to fewer adverse effects and a lower risk of developing drug resistance. Researchers and medical professionals can keep investigating the possibilities of plant compounds as nature's response to viral dangers by utilizing the power of nature's pharmacy.

In summary, focusing on viral entry and replication pathways presents a viable strategy for eradicating viral infections and lessening the impact of viral illnesses on the world's health. Antiviral drugs generated from plants are abundant and possess a variety of modes of action that can effectively impede viral replication and penetration into host cells. Researchers can discover new targets for antiviral medication and create creative ways to fight viral infections by clarifying the molecular mechanisms behind viral entry and reproduction. Furthermore, plant-based antiviral medicines are valuable weapons in the battle against viral threats because of their availability, affordability, and safety. By utilizing plant chemicals' therapeutic potential, we can create efficient plans for treating and preventing viral infections and enhance global population health and wellbeing.

Boosting Immune Response with Plant-Based Compounds

The immune system is essential for protecting the body from viral infections, identifying and getting rid of pathogens, and coordinating the proper immunological response. Improving immune function becomes critical for avoiding and treating infections when faced with viral threats. With their wide range of bioactive chemicals that modify immune function and strengthen antiviral defenses, plant-based drugs have become increasingly important tools for enhancing immunological responses. Using plant components' immunomodulatory capabilities, scientists and medical practitioners can access nature's pharmacy to fortify the body's defenses against viral infections.

Plant-based substances have been shown to partially enhance immunological responses by inducing immune cell activity. The immune system comprises different cell types that cooperate to identify and eradicate pathogens, such as dendritic cells, macrophages, and lymphocytes.

It has been demonstrated that plant-derived substances, such as the polysaccharides present in medicinal mushrooms like reishi (Ganoderma spp.) and astragalus root (Astragalus membranaceus), stimulate immune cell proliferation and activity, improving the body's capacity to mount a successful defense against viral infections. To further strengthen the body's antiviral defenses, polysaccharides can also alter the synthesis of cytokine signaling molecules that control immune responses.

Plant-based substances boost immune cell function and have anti-inflammatory and antioxidant characteristics that lessen the harm caused by viral infections. Viruses frequently cause oxidative stress and inflammation in the tissues they infect, which damages tissue and compromises immune system performance. Flavonoids, plentiful in fruits, vegetables, and herbs, are compounds with potent anti-inflammatory and antioxidant properties that might mitigate the harmful consequences of viral infections. For instance, it has been demonstrated that the flavonoid quercetin, present in citrus fruits, onions, and apples, inhibits the replication of viruses while having antioxidant and anti-inflammatory properties. This improves immune function and lessens the severity of viral infections.

Furthermore, plant-based substances can modify immune responses by controlling the synthesis of inflammatory mediators and cytokines. Over-inflammatory responses can aggravate viral infections and lead to tissue damage. It has been demonstrated that certain compounds, including turmeric, which is extracted from turmeric (Curcuma longa), suppress the generation of pro- inflammatory cytokines while stimulating the creation of anti-inflammatory cytokines. This reduces excessive inflammation and strengthens the immune system. In a similar vein, it has been demonstrated that omega-3 fatty acids, which are present in flaxseeds, walnuts, and fatty fish, can modify immune responses by decreasing the synthesis of pro-inflammatory mediators and encouraging the resolution of inflammation, which strengthens the body's defenses against viral infections.

Additionally, plant substances can strengthen mucosal immunity, which is the body's first line of defense against viral infections at mucosal surfaces, including the gastrointestinal and respiratory systems. It has been demonstrated that substances like flavonoids, present in foods like citrus fruits and green tea, improve the integrity of the mucosal barrier and increase the generation of mucosal antibodies, which stops viruses from entering and spreading across mucosal surfaces. Furthermore, polysaccharides present in medicinal mushrooms, like Grifola frondosa and shiitake (Lentinula edodes), have been demonstrated to activate mucosal immune cells, augmenting mucosal immunity and mitigating the likelihood of viral infections.

Additionally, combining plant-based chemicals can strengthen their immunomodulatory qualities, offering a more comprehensive strategy for enhancing immune responses against viral infections. Traditional herbal treatments are more effective than single compounds because they comprise many plant constituents with complimentary immunomodulatory actions. For instance, traditional medicine has employed the combination of echinacea (Echinacea purpurea) and elderberry (Sambucus nigra) to improve immune function and lessen the intensity and duration of viral infections. Elderberry's antioxidant and antiviral qualities combine with echinacea's stimulation of immune cell activity to offer a comprehensive strategy for enhancing immune responses against viral threats.

Plant-based chemicals are a great way to strengthen antiviral defenses against viral threats and immune responses. Plant chemicals offer a multimodal strategy to fortify the body's resistance against viral infections by inducing immune cell activity, decreasing inflammation, and improving mucosal immunity. Furthermore, plant-based chemicals have synergistic effects and are easily obtainable, making them ideal candidates for developing innovative immunomodulatory medicines to tackle viral infections. Researchers and medical practitioners can use nature's pharmacy to boost immune responses and lessen the impact of viral threats on world health by utilizing the immunomodulatory qualities of plant chemicals.

CHAPTER V

Case Studies and Clinical Evidence

Studies Demonstrating Efficacy of Plant-Based Antivirals

Growing interest has been seen in using plant-based antivirals' therapeutic potential as a natural way to fight viral threats in recent years. Several research investigations have examined the effectiveness of plant chemicals against various types of viruses, presenting strong proof of their antiviral characteristics. These investigations have illuminated the various processes via which plant chemicals exert their antiviral effects, ranging from traditional herbal medicines to contemporary pharmacological research. This has opened up intriguing options for the development of new antiviral therapies.

The antiviral action of polyphenols, a type of bioactive chemical common in fruits, vegetables, and herbs, has been of significant interest to me. Research has demonstrated that polyphenols, such as flavonoids, phenolic acids, and tannins, have strong antiviral properties against various viruses, such as HIV, herpes simplex virus, and influenza. For instance, a research study released in the current issue of the Food and Agricultural Chemistry publication showed that the green tea flavonoid epigallocatechin gallate (EGCG) prevented the influenza virus from replicating by interacting with viral RNA and protein production. Similarly, it has been demonstrated that the flavonoid quercetin, present in onions, apples, and citrus fruits, inhibits the multiplication of respiratory viruses such as influenza and rhinovirus by preventing the virus from entering host cells.

Terpenoids are an additional group of chemicals obtained from plants with antiviral solid characteristics. Terpenoids, which are present in resinous exudates and essential oils of plants, including limonene, eucalyptol, and thymol, have a wide range of antiviral activity against respiratory viruses, herpes simplex virus, and respiratory syncytial virus (RSV). For instance, thymol, a monoterpene phenol present in thyme and other aromatic plants, was shown in a study published in the journal Antiviral Research to impede the reproduction of the herpes simplex virus by interfering with the integrity of viral envelope proteins and the virus's ability to enter host cells. Similarly, it has been demonstrated that the terpenoid eucalyptol present in eucalyptus leaves has strong antiviral properties against influenza viruses by preventing viral reproduction and influencing host immunological responses.

Additionally, the antiviral qualities of alkaloids—
compounds containing nitrogen present in various plant species—have been studied. Research has demonstrated that alkaloids, namely berberine, caffeine, and quinine, have antiviral properties against several infections, which include the human immunodeficiency virus (HIV), herpes simplex virus, and influenza. For instance, berberine, an alkaloid present in goldenseal (Hydrastis canadensis) and other plants, was shown in a study published in Virology to limit influenza virus multiplication by interfering with viral RNA synthesis and protein expression. Similarly, it has been demonstrated that caffeine, a methylxanthine alkaloid present in coffee (Coffea spp.), inhibits the virus that causes herpes simplex virus by interfering with the replication of viral DNA and protein synthesis.

Beta-glucans and mannans, two polysaccharides isolated from plants, have also been studied for their immunomodulatory and antiviral qualities. It has been demonstrated that polysaccharides extracted from medicinal mushrooms, such as reishi (Ganoderma spp.)

and astragalus root (Astragalus membranaceus), boost immunological responses and improve the body's defenses against viral infections. In the journal Phytotherapy Research, a study showed that beta- glucans isolated from reishi mushrooms increased the generation of antiviral cytokines and promoted immune cell activity, decreasing the intensity and duration of respiratory viral infections.

Additionally, many research investigations have demonstrated the effectiveness of plant-based antivirals in treating and preventing viral infections. For instance, the effectiveness of a standardized extract of Pelargonium sidoides root (Umckaloabo) in lowering the severity and length of symptoms in patients with acute respiratory infections brought on by respiratory viruses was a testes-controlled trial that was published in the journal Antimicrobial Agents and Chemotherapy. Comparing patients treated with Pelargonium extract to those getting a placebo, the study revealed that patients' symptoms, including cough, congestion, and sore throat, significantly improved.

In summary, research proving the effectiveness of plant-based antivirals offers strong proof of their potential to be nature's solution to viral threats. Plant-derived polyphenols, terpenoids, alkaloids, and polysaccharides have antiviral solid action against various viruses by influencing the host immune system and selectively targeting different stages of the viral reproduction cycle. Furthermore, scientific trials have demonstrated the effectiveness of plant-based antivirals in treating and preventing viral infections, opening up exciting new possibilities for creating antiviral treatments. Using plant-based antivirals' therapeutic potential, scientists and medical practitioners can investigate novel strategies for battling viral infections and enhancing worldwide health results.

Success Stories of Plant-Based Treatments in Viral Infections

Plant-based remedies have been effectively used to treat viral infections throughout medical history, offering proof of nature's ability to battle viral dangers. Numerous success stories demonstrate the efficacy of plant-based medicines in treating viral infections, ranging from conventional herbal remedies to contemporary pharmaceutical research. These encouraging tales highlight the medicinal value of plants and the significance of looking into nature's pharmacy for cutting- edge antiviral treatments.

One of the most noteworthy achievements in the field of plant-based remedies for viral infections is the identification of quinine, a substance obtained from the cinchona tree's bark, which possesses antiviral characteristics. The drug quinine has been used for centuries to treat malaria, an infectious disease spread by mosquitoes that are brought on by the Plasmodium parasite. Quinine has been shown to have antiviral activity against several viruses, including the human immunodeficiency virus (HIV) and influenza, in addition to its antimalarial properties. This finding made it possible to create synthetic quinine derivatives like chloroquine and hydroxychloroquine, which are now used to treat viral infections like HIV and the virus that caused the COVID-19 pandemic, severe acute respiratory syndrome coronavirus 2 (SARS-CoV-2).

Tamiflu, also known as oseltamivir, is a plant-based influenza medication that has proven effective in treating viral infections. This medication is an inhibitor of the neuraminidase enzyme that influenza viruses manufacture. It is created from shikimic acid, a chemical that grows in the star anise plant (Illicium verum).

Oseltamivir decreases the propagation of the virus

throughout the body by preventing the release of freshly generated viral particles from infected host cells by inhibiting neuraminidase activity. When given early in the course of the infection, oseltamivir, a commonly used front-line treatment for influenza, is beneficial in lowering the severity and duration of symptoms.

Additionally, traditional herbal therapies utilized by indigenous societies worldwide successfully treat viral infections when derived from plants. For example, several traditional medical systems, such as European herbalism and Native American medicine, have documented elderberry (Sambucus spp.) as a therapy for respiratory infections. Bioactive substances found in elderberries, such as flavonoids and anthocyanins, have antiviral qualities by preventing the growth of viruses and influencing the body's defense mechanisms. Clinical research has demonstrated that elderberry extract is a valuable adjunct to natural treatments for viral illnesses, as it helps lessen the intensity and duration of symptoms in individuals suffering from influenza and other respiratory infections.

Furthermore, herbal formulations used in traditional Chinese medicine (TCM) are an excellent example of how well plant-based medicines work in treating viral infections. Traditional Chinese medicine (TCM) practitioners have used a range of herbal medicines for ages to treat viral illnesses, including herpes simplex virus, hepatitis, and influenza. One well-known instance is using Andrographis paniculata, or just Andrographis, to treat respiratory infections. Bioactive substances in andrographis, such as andrographolides, have immune-stimulating solid and antiviral properties. Andrographis extract is a standard treatment for viral respiratory disorders in traditional Chinese medicine (TCM) therapy because clinical studies have demonstrated that it can lessen the intensity and duration of symptoms in individuals with upper respiratory tract infections.

Furthermore, current pharmacological research has revealed novel antiviral chemicals originating from plants, supporting the efficacy of plant-based medicines in treating viral infections. For instance, research into EGCG—a polyphenol present in green tea (Camellia sinensis)—as a possible therapy for viral infections, including the flu and human papillomavirus (HPV), has been prompted by the polyphenol's antiviral qualities. EGCG is a good option for creating innovative antiviral treatments because it has been demonstrated to suppress viral replication and alter immune responses. Comparably, research into berberine—an alkaloid present in goldenseal (Hydrastis canadensis) and other plants—as a possible remedy for viral illnesses including hepatitis B virus (HBV) and herpes simplex virus (HSV) has been spurred by the alkaloid's antiviral qualities. Inhibiting viral replication and lowering inflammation, berberine is a valuable addition to natural treatments for viral illnesses.

In summary, the success stories of using plants to cure viral infections demonstrate the medicinal potential of plants as the body's natural defense against viral threats. Plants have long been essential sources of resources for the fight against viral infections, from historical herbal medicines to contemporary pharmacological research. Using chemicals derived from plants with antiviral capabilities, scientists and medical practitioners can further investigate novel methods for controlling viral infections and enhancing worldwide health results.

Potential Applications in Various Viral Diseases

Numerous resources found in nature have the potential to be effective in the fight against a wide range of viruses that cause viral illnesses. Naturally occurring chemicals have a wide range of potential applications in treating different viral infections, ranging from current pharmaceutical research to traditional herbal therapies.

These natural remedies offer accessible and long-lasting ways to combat viral dangers across the globe in addition to providing efficient therapies. By investigating the possible uses of nature's response to viral threats, we can find new ways to control viral diseases and enhance the state of global health.

Care of respiratory viral infections, such as influenza, respiratory syncytial virus (RSV), and coronaviruses like severe acute respiratory syndrome coronavirus 2 (SARS-CoV-2), is one area where natural remedies hold great promise. Compounded with polyphenols, terpenoids, and polysaccharides, traditional herbal treatments have shown strong antiviral effectiveness against respiratory viruses through the suppression of viral reproduction, adjustment of immunological responses, and improvement of mucosal immunity. Examples of compounds that show promise for developing natural treatments for respiratory diseases include quercetin from fruits and vegetables and epigallocatechin gallate (EGCG) from green tea. These compounds have been shown to inhibit viral replication and reduce inflammation in respiratory viral infections.

Additionally, there is hope for the treatment of sexually transmitted illnesses like HIV, herpes simplex virus, and human papillomavirus (HSV) with natural remedies. Compounds originating from plants, including lignans, alkaloids, and flavonoids, have shown antiviral action against sexually transmitted infections by modifying immune responses, preventing viral entry into host cells, and suppressing viral reproduction. For instance, it has been demonstrated that substances like berberine from goldenseal and curcumin from turmeric prevent HPV and HSV from replicating, and they also have immune-stimulating properties that may help manage HIV infection.

Moreover, natural remedies have the potential to be used in the management of rotavirus, hepatitis, and norovirus infections of the gastrointestinal tract. Plant-derived substances such as polysaccharides, lignans, and tannins have been shown to have antiviral efficacy against gastrointestinal viruses through their ability to enhance mucosal immunity, prevent viral entry into host cells, and limit viral replication. Certain substances, such as lignans from flaxseeds and ellagic acid from berries, have been demonstrated to have gastroprotective properties that may help manage hepatitis viruses and to limit the reproduction of rotavirus and norovirus.

Furthermore, natural remedies have the potential to treat viral diseases that insects like ticks and mosquitoes spread. Plant-derived substances such as terpenoids, alkaloids, and pyrethrins have shown antiviral efficacy against viruses that enter host cells through their ability to impede viral replication and reject or eliminate disease vectors. For instance, it has been demonstrated that substances like pyrethrins from chrysanthemum flowers and quassinoids from quassia bark inhibit the reproduction of viruses carried by mosquitoes, including the Zika and dengue viruses. These compounds also possess insecticidal qualities that may aid in the management of disease vectors and the prevention of viral disease transmission.

In addition, natural remedies may be used in the management of viral meningitis, West Nile virus encephalitis, herpes simplex encephalitis, and other viral disorders impacting the central nervous system (CNS). Plant-derived substances such as flavonoids, alkaloids, and terpenoids have shown antiviral efficacy against central nervous system (CNS) viruses by influencing immune responses inside the central nervous system, preventing viral reproduction in neural cells, and overcoming the blood-brain barrier. For instance, it has been demonstrated that substances like hypericin from

St. John's wort and ginkgolides from the herb ginkgo biloba inhibit the growth of the West Nile and herpes simplex viruses in neural cells while also displaying neuroprotective properties that may help treat meningitis and viral encephalitis.

In summary, there are a plethora of possible uses for nature's response to viral threats, including a broad spectrum of viral illnesses that impact distinct organ systems and routes of transmission. Natural chemicals produced from plants offer intriguing solutions for addressing viral threats globally, ranging from gastrointestinal and vector-borne diseases to respiratory and STDs. Researchers and medical professionals might keep investigating novel strategies for controlling viral infections and enhancing the state of worldwide health by utilizing nature's pharmacy. Nature's remedies have the power to transform antiviral therapy and offer efficient, affordable, and long-lasting medicines for viral illnesses with additional study and advancement.

CHAPTER VI

Harvesting and Processing Plant-Based Antivirals

Sustainable Sourcing Practices

The need for sustainable sourcing strategies in utilizing nature's resources to counteract the growing threat of viral diseases is becoming increasingly apparent. Sustainable sourcing is the ethical acquisition of natural resources and ingredients with the least detrimental effects on the environment and society. Sustainable sourcing procedures are essential for guaranteeing the availability, quality, and ethical manufacturing of plant-based treatments and natural substances utilized in antiviral therapy in the context of nature's response to viral threats. Researchers, medical practitioners, and businesses may optimize the advantages of nature's medicine while preserving biodiversity, ecosystems, and nearby populations by implementing sustainable sourcing procedures.

Promoting biodiversity conservation and protection is a central tenet of sustainable sourcing techniques. Many plant species utilized in natural medicine systems and traditional herbal medicines are taken from wild populations, which puts them at risk of overuse and depletion. By encouraging the production of medicinal plants in regulated settings like botanical gardens, nurseries, and agroforestry systems, sustainable sourcing approaches seek to reduce these hazards. It is feasible to reduce pressure on wild populations, preserve biodiversity, and guarantee plant-based treatments' long-term availability to fend off viral threats by growing medicinal plants sustainably.

Furthermore, maintaining natural ecosystems and habitats for the growth of medicinal plants is a top priority for sustainable sourcing techniques. Significant risks to biodiversity and ecosystem integrity include habitat degradation, deforestation, and land conversion for agriculture. These actions result in plant species extinction and disturbance of natural processes. Sustainable sourcing techniques support habitat conservation, reforestation, and sustainable land management to preserve and restore natural ecosystems. The ecological balance can be upheld, biodiversity conservation can be supported, and the habitats of medicinal plants vital to antiviral treatments can be protected by protecting natural environments.

Additionally, the ethical treatment of nearby populations and indigenous peoples—who rely on medicinal plants for their livelihoods and traditional customs—is emphasized by sustainable sourcing procedures. Many traditional medical systems have origins in generations-old indigenous knowledge and customs. However, the commercial use of medicinal herbs frequently results in the marginalization, exploitation, and cultural appropriation of indigenous people. Fair benefit distribution, adherence to indigenous rights, and community involvement in decisions about procuring and applying medicinal plants are prioritized in sustainable sourcing procedures. It is possible to guarantee that the advantages of nature's resources are distributed fairly and that indigenous knowledge and cultural practices are maintained and conserved by cultivating partnerships with local populations.

Sustainable sourcing methods also support open supply chains and traceability programs to guarantee the integrity and caliber of natural chemicals and plant-based medicines. Concerns regarding adulteration, contamination, and mislabeling of herbal treatments and botanical extracts have arisen due to trade globalization and the demand for natural products. Sustainable sourcing methods encourage accountability and openness at every stage of the supply chain, from production and harvesting to distribution and processing. Plant-based medicines can have their safety, efficacy, and little risk of side effects confirmed by using quality control and traceability mechanisms to ensure their authenticity and safety.

Additionally, the utilization of socially and environmentally responsible production techniques in the growing, harvesting, and processing medicinal plants is given top priority in sustainable sourcing processes. Some examples of sustainable production techniques that minimize synthetic inputs, lessen environmental impacts, and support fair labor practices are organic farming, agroecological practices, and fair-trade activities. Using sustainable production techniques can help reduce pollution, preserve the ecosystem, and promote the welfare of the communities and laborers who produce plant-based medicines.

To sum up, to successfully and ethically tackle viral risks, it is imperative to implement sustainable sourcing procedures. To optimize the benefits of plant-based medicines while preserving ecosystems, biodiversity, and local communities, adopting environmentally friendly production practices, respecting indigenous rights, conserving natural habitats, promoting biodiversity conservation, ensuring transparency and traceability, and protecting biodiversity is possible. Adopting sustainable sourcing procedures is essential as the globe struggles with the persistent problems caused by viral infections. This will guarantee nature's pharmacy's long-term availability, effectiveness, and moral application in combating viral threats.

Extraction Methods for Maximum Potency

Selecting the proper extraction techniques is essential to enhancing the potency and effectiveness of natural chemicals and plant-based therapies in the fight against viral threats. This is part of the effort to maximize the therapeutic potential of nature's pharmacy. The processes used to separate bioactive molecules from plant sources and concentrate their medicinal qualities for therapeutic application are called extraction methods. Various extraction techniques—including more contemporary approaches like solvent extraction, supercritical fluid extraction, and more conventional ones like maceration and decoction—offer clear advantages to extracting bioactive compounds with antiviral characteristics. Using extraction techniques that maximize bioactive substances' quantity, quality, and stability, scientists and medical experts can fully explore the therapeutic possibilities of nature's response to virus hazards.

Herbal medicines and medicinal tinctures have been made for ages using conventional extraction techniques, including maceration and decoction. Plant materials are macerated by soaking in a solvent, like alcohol or water, to release bioactive chemicals through diffusion. Plant materials are boiled in water during the decoction process to extract heat-stable components, including tannins and polysaccharides, which may have antiviral qualities.

Traditional extraction techniques are easy to use and reasonably priced. However, they only sometimes produce high quantities of bioactive substances. They might only be able to extract specific classes of compounds, including alkaloids and volatile oils, to a limited extent. However, these techniques are still helpful in isolating a wide range of bioactive substances from therapeutic plants, and they have played a crucial role in creating conventional herbal treatments for viral infections.

Modern extraction methods, such as supercritical fluid and solvent extraction, have advantages in terms of extracting particular classes of very potent and pure bioactive chemicals. Utilizing organic solvents like ethanol or methanol, solvent extraction entails dissolving bioactive chemicals from plant materials and then evaporating the extract to concentrate them. Alkaloids and essential oils are lipophilic substances that can be effectively extracted using this technique and have strong antiviral properties. On the other hand, supercritical fluid extraction uses high-pressure and temperature supercritical fluids—like carbon dioxide—to extract non- polar and semi-polar chemicals from plant materials. This technique minimizes the need for organic solvents. It protects the integrity of heat-sensitive molecules while enabling the selective extraction of particular bioactive components. Researchers can precisely control the extraction parameters using solvent extraction and supercritical fluid extraction. This enables them to maximize the production and potency of bioactive molecules for antiviral treatments.

Additionally, cutting-edge extraction methods like microwave- and ultrasound-assisted extraction have become viable strategies for raising the effectiveness and speed of extraction procedures. Comparing ultrasound-assisted extraction to conventional approaches, higher extraction yields and shorter extraction periods are achieved by using high-frequency sound waves to break down cell walls and improve the release of bioactive chemicals from plant materials. By using microwave radiation to create heat and improve mass transfer and diffusion, microwave-assisted extraction makes it easier to extract bioactive chemicals. These novel extraction methods' effectiveness, repeatability, and sustainability make them valuable instruments for extracting bioactive substances with antiviral qualities from therapeutic plants.

Furthermore, the potency and effectiveness of plant-based treatments for viral infections can significantly impact the choice of extraction solvents and circumstances. Since different types of bioactive chemicals have differing solvent solubilities, choosing suitable extraction solvents to target particular compounds of interest requires careful thought. The quantity and makeup of extracted compounds can also be influenced by temperature, pressure, and extraction duration; the ideal parameters will vary based on the type of plant and the desired compounds. Through methodical optimization of extraction settings, scientists can optimize the effectiveness and potency of plant-based therapies in the fight against viral threats.

Extraction techniques are essential for optimizing the strength and effectiveness of natural chemicals and plant-based medicines against viral threats. Bioactive compounds with antiviral qualities can be facilitated by modern techniques like supercritical fluid extraction and solvent extraction, as well as by more traditional procedures like maceration and decoction. The efficiency and speed of extraction operations are further improved by cutting-edge techniques like ultrasound- and microwave-assisted extraction, enabling researchers to realize the medicinal potential of nature's pharmacy fully. Through meticulous selection of extraction techniques and optimization of extraction parameters, scientists and medical practitioners can leverage the potential of nature's response to viral hazards and create efficacious therapies for viral illnesses.

Ensuring Quality and Safety Standards

Both conventional and contemporary medicine can combat viral threats and treat infectious diseases by utilizing nature's pharmacy. Traditional medicinal systems based on indigenous knowledge and practices have traditionally treated viral infections using herbal remedies and natural ingredients. Modern medicine, on the other hand, makes use of cutting-edge tools, exacting testing protocols, and scientific investigation. Scientists, doctors, and legislators may create comprehensive programs to prevent viral risks and maintain the efficacy, safety, and accessibility of pharmaceuticals by combining the advantages of both systems.

There is a lot of information available regarding the use of herbal medicines and medicinal plants to treat viral infections in traditional medical systems including Ayurveda, Traditional Chinese Medicine (TCM), and Indigenous healing practices. Encounters challenges as a result of viral infections. People have been using herbal remedies containing bioactive compounds, such as polyphenols, flavonoids, alkaloids, and terpenoids, for millennia to reduce inflammation, boost immunity, and halt the spread of infections. For example, viral illnesses have been treated in India using Ayurvedic herbs, including Holy Basil and Andrographis paniculata. In the meantime, Chinese traditional medicine has long employed TCM formulations such as Yin Qiao San and Ma Huang Tang to treat viral infections of the respiratory system. Scientists can identify natural chemicals and plant-based medicines that show potential for further investigation and development by leveraging the knowledge of traditional medical systems.

Traditional knowledge is complemented by scientific rigor, technological innovation, and evidence-based pharmaceutical discovery and development procedures in modern medicine. From plant extracts and natural products that may have antiviral qualities, scientists can extract bioactive compounds using advanced techniques, including molecular modeling, high-throughput screening, and bioinformatics. Furthermore, modern analytical methods such as mass spectrometry, chromatography, and nuclear magnetic resonance (NMR) spectroscopy make it easier to isolate, characterize, and purify bioactive chemicals. This makes it possible to evaluate these substances pharmacologically and conduct clinical trials. By applying contemporary medical methodologies and techniques, researchers can verify the safety, effectiveness, and mechanisms of action of plant-based medicines. This will make it easier to incorporate these treatments into traditional medical practice.

Conventional and contemporary medicine collaborate outside of the laboratory through clinical research, patient care, and public health initiatives. Clinical trials provide vital information to support the use of traditional herbal remedies for viral infections in contemporary healthcare settings by assessing their safety and effectiveness. Integrative medicine, which combines complementary and alternative therapies, offers patients with viral illnesses complete, tailored therapy. Additionally, communities all around the world benefit from public health campaigns that support the use of plant-based medications for preventative healthcare, such as immune-boosting herbal supplements and teas.

Cooperation between traditional and modern medicine also fosters respect for one another, the development of ability, and the exchange of knowledge among practitioners and different healthcare systems. Interdisciplinary research collaborations bring scientists, herbalists, pharmacists, and clinicians together to share information, resources, and best practices in medicine creation, formulation, and clinical treatment. Additionally, initiatives to document and conserve traditional knowledge, such as ethnobotanical surveys and databases for traditional medicine, promote respect for indigenous healing practices and a greater understanding of cultural variety. Stakeholders can work together to address global health concerns and improve healthcare outcomes by promoting dialogue and cooperation between traditional and modern medicine.

The successful collaboration of traditional and contemporary medicine requires adherence to ethical considerations and cultural sensitivity. It is imperative to uphold the rights of indigenous peoples, intellectual property, and cultural heritage in order to establish equitable partnerships that benefit all stakeholders. Initiatives that promote inclusivity, diversity, and cultural competence in healthcare procedures also facilitate successful communication and collaboration between patients, medical staff, and traditional healers. By working together, we can eliminate viral threats and improve health and well-being for future generations while also valuing cultural diversity and traditional medicinal systems.

In short, harnessing nature's pharmacy to combat viral threats through a fusion of traditional and modern treatment has great promise. Scholars, doctors, and legislators can develop new methods for identifying, treating, and preventing viral infections by fusing modern science with traditional knowledge. In addition to ensuring the safety, effectiveness, and cultural sensitivity of healthcare interventions, collaboration fosters ethical behavior and mutual respect for one another's cultures. Even as the world struggles with viral infections, collaborative initiatives between traditional and modern medicine provide hope for a healthier, more resilient future.

CHAPTER VII

Integrating Plant-Based Antivirals into Healthcare

Collaboration between Traditional and Modern Medicine

Traditional and modern medicine can battle viral threats and use nature's pharmacy to fight infectious diseases. Herbal treatments and natural substances have long been used by traditional medical systems rooted in indigenous knowledge and practices to treat viral infections. On the other hand, modern medicine uses cutting-edge technologies, rigorous testing procedures, and scientific research. Researchers, medical professionals, and legislators can create complete strategies for combating viral dangers while guaranteeing the efficacy, safety, and accessibility of medicines by fusing the advantages of both approaches.

A wealth of information about applying natural remedies and medicinal plants to treat viral infections may be found in traditional medicine systems, including Ayurveda, Traditional Chinese Medicine (TCM), and Indigenous healing customs. For millennia, people have utilized herbal treatments that include bioactive substances, including polyphenols, flavonoids, alkaloids, and terpenoids, to suppress inflammation, increase immunity, and stop the spread of viruses. For instance, Ayurvedic herbs like Andrographis paniculata and Holy Basil have been utilized in India to treat viral disorders. At the same time, TCM formulations like Yin Qiao San and Ma Huang Tang have been used traditionally in China to treat respiratory viral infections. By utilizing the knowledge of conventional medical systems, scientists can pinpoint natural substances and plant-based treatments that show promise for more research and development.

Scientific rigor, technological innovation, and evidence-based medication discovery and development approaches complement modern medicine with traditional wisdom. Using sophisticated methods like molecular modeling, high-throughput screening, and bioinformatics, scientists can extract bioactive chemicals from plant extracts and natural products that may have antiviral properties. Furthermore, bioactive compounds' isolation, characterization, and purification are more accessible by contemporary analytical techniques, including nuclear magnetic resonance (NMR) spectroscopy, mass spectrometry, and chromatography. This enables the pharmacological assessment and clinical testing of these compounds. Researchers can validate plant-based treatments' safety, efficacy, and mechanisms of action by utilizing modern medical methods and techniques. This will facilitate the integration of these remedies into mainstream healthcare.

Collaboration between clinical research, patient care, and public health efforts is where traditional and modern medicine work together outside the laboratory. Clinical trials offer essential data to support the use of traditional herbal treatments in contemporary healthcare settings by assessing their safety and effectiveness in treating viral infections. Patients with viral disorders can receive comprehensive and individualized care through integrative medicine, blending traditional remedies with conventional treatments. Furthermore, public health initiatives that support using plant-based medicines for preventive healthcare—like immune-boosting herbal supplements and teas—help communities worldwide prevent sickness and promote good health.

Furthermore, conventional and modern medicine cooperation promotes mutual respect, capacity building, and knowledge sharing among various healthcare systems and practitioners. To exchange knowledge, resources, and best practices in medication development, formulation, and clinical management, interdisciplinary research collaborations bring together scientists, herbalists, pharmacists, and clinicians. Moreover, programs like ethnobotanical surveys and traditional medicine databases that work to preserve and record traditional knowledge foster respect for indigenous healing customs and a deeper appreciation of cultural diversity. To address global health issues and enhance healthcare results, stakeholders can cooperate by encouraging communication and collaboration between traditional and modern medicine.

Ethical issues and cultural sensitivity are essential for traditional and contemporary medicine to collaborate successfully. Respect for indigenous rights, intellectual property, and cultural heritage is crucial to ensure fair relationships and benefits for all parties involved. Furthermore, initiatives that support diversity, inclusivity, and cultural competence in healthcare practices help patients, healthcare professionals, and traditional healers collaborate and communicate effectively. Collaborative approaches that acknowledge the value of traditional medicine systems and value cultural variety can harness human expertise to combat viral dangers and advance health and well-being for future generations.

In summary, combining traditional and modern medicine has enormous potential for using nature's pharmacy to fight viral threats. By integrating contemporary scientific research with traditional knowledge, scholars, medical practitioners, and policymakers can create novel approaches to preventing, diagnosing, and treating viral infections. Collaboration also promotes ethical behavior, respect for one another's cultures, and cultural sensitivity, guaranteeing healthcare interventions' efficacy, safety, and cultural sensitivity. Collaborative efforts between traditional and modern medicine give hope for a healthier, more resilient future, even as the globe faces difficulties from viral infections.

Challenges and Opportunities in Integrating Plant- Based Therapies

The addition of plant-based therapeutics to the defense against viral threats poses opportunities and obstacles in the search for comprehensive and efficient medical treatments. Due to its many therapeutic benefits, plant-based therapies—which come from natural sources, including herbs, medicinal plants, and botanical extracts —have been used for centuries in traditional medical systems throughout the world. Due to their extensive repertoire of bioactive chemicals with antiviral action, these medicines present intriguing possibilities for the treatment of viral infections. Plant-based medicines do, however, confront several obstacles in their mainstream healthcare integration, including regulatory permission, standardization, acceptance in the community, and scientific confirmation. Notwithstanding these obstacles, there are plenty of chances to take advantage of the potential of plant-based therapeutics to support traditional medical care and advance international initiatives to combat viral threats.

The requirement for solid scientific data to demonstrate the safety and efficacy of plant-based medicines for viral threats is one of the main obstacles to their integration. Traditional medical systems have historically guided therapeutic practices with empirical observations and anecdotal evidence; nevertheless, modern healthcare requires rigorous scientific validation through preclinical and clinical research. Determining the best dose schedules and understanding the mechanisms of action of herbal treatments are difficult due to their complexity since they contain a variety of bioactive components with distinct pharmacological effects. Standardized protocols and quality control techniques are necessary to assure the repeatability and dependability of results in scientific research, as the variety in plant content, growing conditions, and extraction processes add a layer of complexity.

Another obstacle to mainstreaming plant-based medicines in healthcare is regulatory approval, which varies depending on the jurisdiction and its norms and structure. There are disparities in quality, safety, and efficacy between nations because some have set up regulatory channels for the registration and marketing authorization of herbal medicines and natural products. In contrast, others need more regulatory control or defined rules. Plant-based therapy approval processes might be streamlined by harmonizing regulatory standards and allowing mutual recognition agreements. This would enable the therapies to enter international markets and guarantee uniform quality and safety standards for customers around the globe.

Because changes in plant composition, extraction processes, and formulation procedures can result in variability in potency and efficacy, standardizing herbal medicines and botanical extracts is a substantial barrier to maintaining consistency and quality control. Standardization entails creating standards for the recognition, validation, and measurement of bioactive substances in herbal products and guaranteeing uniformity in production and quality control procedures. To standardize herbal medications and confirm their composition, purity, and stability, sophisticated analytical techniques such as spectroscopy, molecular profiling, and chromatography are crucial. Manufacturers can guarantee the dependability and consistency of plant-based treatments for viral risks by implementing standardized procedures and quality control systems.

Using plant-based treatments to combat viral threats presents extra problems related to cultural acceptance and integration into mainstream healthcare systems. Although many cultures and communities have long considered traditional medical systems essential to their healthcare practices, their incorporation into contemporary healthcare systems may encounter opposition, mistrust, and cultural hurdles. Patients' and healthcare providers' acceptance of herbal therapies may be hampered by misconceptions regarding their efficacy, safety, and legitimacy, as well as worries about possible interactions with conventional medications. Education, communication, and mutual respect for various healing traditions are necessary to close the gap between traditional and modern medicine. Multidisciplinary collaboration between practitioners of various healthcare modalities is also encouraged.

Notwithstanding these obstacles, noteworthy prospects exist for incorporating plant-based treatments into the combat against viral hazards, capitalizing on their varied pharmacological characteristics and cultural significance.

Herbal medicines with bioactive ingredients like terpenoids, alkaloids, polyphenols, and flavonoids have shown antiviral solid action against viral infections, such as coronaviruses, influenza, and retroviruses.

Additionally, herbal remedies address the drawbacks of traditional antiviral medications, such as drug resistance, side effects, and limited effectiveness against newly emerging virus strains. These alternatives and supplements provide complementary and alternative therapy choices for viral infections.

Additionally, there are chances to increase study, funding, and innovation in plant-based treatments for viral risks due to the increased interest in holistic and natural approaches to healthcare. Novel antiviral chemicals and formulations are being discovered due to the therapeutic potential of medicinal plants and botanical extracts being unlocked by advances in pharmacognosy, phytochemistry, and ethnobotany. Furthermore, patients with viral diseases can receive individualized and comprehensive care alternatives from integrative medicine techniques focusing on their mental, spiritual, and physical health. These approaches blend traditional therapies with conventional treatments.

To fully realize the promise of plant-based medicines in combating viral threats, cooperation between herbalists, scientists, policymakers, and traditional healers is required. The divide between conventional and modern medicine can be closed through interdisciplinary research collaborations, knowledge-sharing forums, and capacity-building programs that promote cooperation, mutual respect, and understanding. Additionally, community outreach, education, and public health campaigns can increase knowledge of the advantages of plant-based treatments for viral infections, encouraging acceptance and incorporation of these treatments into conventional medical procedures.

In conclusion, there are many chances to take advantage of plant-based medicines' therapeutic potential to improve global health outcomes, even though incorporating them into the battle against viral threats presents particular challenges. To fully realize the potential of plant-based therapeutics for viral infections, overcoming specific difficulties and obtaining regulatory permission, standardization, cultural acceptance, and scientific validation will be necessary. Stakeholders can use the collective understanding of current scientific research and traditional medical systems to develop safe, effective, and culturally relevant remedies for viral threats by promoting collaboration, creativity, and cultural sensitivity. Despite the world's continued struggles with viral infections, using plant-based treatments gives hope for a more robust and healthy future.

Future Directions and Research Needs

While viral threats continue to pose unprecedented problems to the world, there is great potential in exploring nature's pharmacy for antiviral medicines. Natural medicines derived from plants and other materials provide abundant bioactive chemicals that can potentially treat various viral diseases. However, future research efforts must tackle significant hurdles, expand scientific understanding, and turn findings into practical treatments to fully harness the therapeutic potential of nature's response to viral threats. Researchers, medical professionals, and legislators can open the door for novel approaches to battle viral illnesses and improve global health outcomes by identifying future paths and research needs.

Clarifying the mechanisms of action of bioactive substances from medicinal plants and natural products is one of the main topics of future research in nature's response to viral threats. Although numerous drugs originating from plants have shown antiviral solid activity in preclinical investigations, little is known about their exact mechanisms of action. More research is required to fully comprehend how these substances interact with host cell receptors, immunological signaling pathways, and viral proteins to produce their antiviral effects. By clarifying the modes of action of bioactive chemicals, scientists can find new targets for drug discovery and improve our knowledge of the host-virus relationship and viral pathogenesis.

Furthermore, future investigations should focus on identifying and synthesizing novel antiviral substances in nature's pharmacy from unexplored sources. There is still much to learn about the variety of plant species and their possible therapeutic uses, even though traditional herbal treatments have long been employed for their medical qualities. Discovering new plant species and natural products with solid antiviral properties can come from investigating uncharted ecosystems, biodiversity hotspots, and conventional medical systems. Furthermore, new developments in high-throughput screening, bioprospecting, and bioinformatics present chances to speed up the identification of novel antiviral agents derived from natural sources. Researchers can overcome obstacles like medication resistance and viral diversity and increase the number of antiviral medicines available by utilizing nature's pharmacy.

Moreover, future research endeavors should optimize the formulation, transport, and pharmacokinetics of natural substances and plant-based treatments for antiviral therapy. Many plant-derived chemicals' low bioavailability, stability, and solubility can restrict their medicinal potential and usefulness. The pharmacokinetic qualities of plant-based medicines can be improved by liposomal administration, nanoencapsulation, and prodrug design, increasing the drugs' absorption, distribution, and retention in the intended tissues. Additionally, new developments in drug delivery technology, such as implantable devices, inhalable nanoparticles, and microneedle patches, provide creative ways to release antiviral chemicals in a targeted and sustained manner.

Through the optimization of formulation and delivery systems, scientists can surmount efficacy constraints and augment the therapeutic potential of plant-based remedies for viral infections.

Future studies should focus on assessing plant-based treatments' pharmacological interactions, safety, and effectiveness in medical contexts. Although preclinical research has demonstrated the potential of many plant-derived substances, human trials must rigorously evaluate these molecules before they may be used in clinical settings. To provide solid evidence for the use of plant-based medicines for viral infections in mainstream healthcare In addition, post-marketing surveillance and pharmacovigilance studies are required to watch for any possible adverse effects, drug interactions, and long-term safety issues related to plant-based therapies. Through well-planned pharmacovigilance and clinical trials, scientists can guarantee the secure and efficient incorporation of plant-based treatments into medical practice.

Subsequent investigations should focus on resolving inequalities in the availability of plant-based treatments and advocating for their fair allocation and application around the globe. Although many cultures and societies have long incorporated traditional medicine systems into their healthcare practices, access to plant-based medicines is still restricted for marginalized populations such as native peoples, rural communities, and low-income nations. Plant-based medicines can be made more accessible and affordable by supporting local production, sustainable agriculture, and community empowerment. Plant-based remedies can also be included in national healthcare policies and programs with the help of initiatives to incorporate traditional medicine into mainstream healthcare systems. These initiatives include training programs for healthcare professionals and the regulatory recognition of traditional healers.

To sum up, a variety of areas require further research to fully understand nature's response to viral threats, including mechanistic investigations, medication discovery, formulation optimization, clinical evaluation, and equitable access. Researchers, medical professionals, and policymakers may fully realize the potential of plant-based treatments in the fight against viral infections and in promoting global health outcomes by tackling these critical issues and expanding scientific knowledge. Realizing the potential of nature's pharmacy as a source of potent medicines for viral threats and advancing this subject will require cooperation, creativity, and interdisciplinary approaches. Investing in the research and development of plant-based treatments is essential for enhancing sustainability, readiness, and resilience against future pandemics and infectious illnesses as the globe continues to face viral threats.

CHAPTER VIII

DIY Herbal Remedies and Recipes

Simple Herbal Preparations for Antiviral Support

Essential herbal remedies are a significant means of bolstering the body's defenses against viral threats and preventing infectious diseases. Since ancient times, traditional medical systems worldwide have used herbal remedies, which are made from medicinal plants and botanical extracts, for their many therapeutic benefits, including antiviral activity. People can boost their immune systems to ward against viral infections and supplement traditional therapies using nature's pharmacy. Plant-based therapies can be easily incorporated into everyday healthcare routines using simple herbal preparations, including steam inhalations, poultices, tinctures, and herbal teas. These methods promote overall wellbeing, which is an economical and accessible option for antiviral support.

Herbal teas, made by steeping fresh or dried medicinal herbs in hot water to release their therapeutic ingredients, are among the most accessible and widely available herbal remedies for antiviral therapy. Herbs with immune-boosting and antiviral qualities, like licorice root, ginger, peppermint, elderberry, and echinacea, are frequently used in herbal teas. Elderberry tea is high in antioxidants and has been demonstrated to block viral replication. In contrast, echinacea tea is well-known for its capacity to boost the immune system and lessen the intensity and length of viral illnesses. People can naturally assist their bodies against viral dangers while hydrating, nourishing, and fortifying them by including herbal teas in their daily routines.

Herbal tinctures, which provide a strong dosage of therapeutic plant extracts in a little liquid form, can provide a concentrated and practical type of herbal medicine. Traditionally, tinctures are made by macerating medicinal herbs in glycerin or alcohol to extract their active ingredients. This process yields a concentrated liquid extract capable of being consumed straight from the container or mixed into other drinks. As tinctures, herbs with antiviral, antibacterial, and immune-stimulating qualities, like garlic, echinacea, oregano, and thyme, are frequently utilized. For instance, echinacea tincture is high in immune-stimulating polysaccharides and alkylamides. In contrast, garlic tincture contains allicin, a substance with strong antiviral properties. People can personalize their antiviral support and strengthen their resistance to infectious diseases by adding herbal tinctures to their routines.

Topical herbal therapies, such as poultices and compresses, provide targeted comfort, antiviral support for skin and respiratory diseases, and oral preparations. A compress is applied to the skin after a cloth has been soaked in a herbal infusion or decoction. In contrast, a poultice is prepared by applying a paste or mixture of crushed herbs directly to the affected area. Calendula, eucalyptus, lavender, and tea tree oil are popular herbs used in compresses and poultices because of their anti-inflammatory, antibacterial, and wound-healing qualities.

For instance, calendula poultices help mend and relieve skin irritations, and eucalyptus compresses are good for clearing sinusitis and lung congestion. Topical herbal medicines can treat viral symptoms and aid the body's natural healing processes as part of self-care regimens.

Additionally, inhaling steam infused with aromatic herbs can help with congestion and respiratory infections by providing antiviral effects and respiratory support. Steam inhalations use fresh or dried herbs—such as thyme, peppermint, rosemary, or eucalyptus—added to hot water to open up the airways, reduce congestion, and support respiratory health. The antibacterial, expectorant, and decongestant volatile oils found in these herbs help to relieve the symptoms of viral respiratory infections, including the flu, bronchitis, and colds. For instance, peppermint includes menthol, which helps to calm irritated airways and lessen coughing. At the same time, eucalyptus has cineole, a chemical with antiviral and mucolytic characteristics. People can reduce their symptoms of respiratory viral infections and expedite their recovery by adding steam inhalations into their regular routines.

Herbal baths can provide a calming and therapeutic means of boosting immunity, enhancing general wellbeing, and providing antiviral assistance. To relieve aching muscles, relax the mind, and strengthen immunity, take an herbal bath by combining fresh or dried herbs like thyme, lavender, rosemary, or chamomile with warm water. These herbs' antiviral, anti-inflammatory, and stress-relieving aromatic components make them perfect for boosting immunity and promoting relaxation.

For example, chamomile and lavender contain flavonoids with immune-boosting qualities and linalool, which has antiviral and anxiolytic effects. People can encourage relaxation, lessen stress, and bolster their resistance to viral dangers by including herbal baths in their self-care regimens.

In conclusion, essential herbal medicines provide easy-to-use, reasonably priced, and efficient methods to bolster the body's natural defenses and counteract viral threats. In everyday healthcare, plant-based therapies can be adaptable to herbal teas, tinctures, poultices, steam inhalations, and herbal baths that enhance overall wellbeing and antimicrobial support. People can boost their immune systems, fortify their defenses against infectious diseases, and supplement traditional medical treatments by utilizing nature's pharmacy. Simple herbal remedies provide a natural and comprehensive way to assist everyone's health and wellbeing as wellbeing struggles with virus outbreaks.

Safety Considerations and Dosage Guidelines

The growing interest in using nature's pharmacy to fight viral threats necessitates the establishment of dosage guidelines and careful examination of safety issues in order to guarantee the safe and efficient use of plant-based medicines. Although natural chemicals and medicinal plants have great promise to combat viral infections, improper use can result in toxicity, negative interactions with drugs, and other hazards. Therefore, optimizing the advantages of nature's response to viral threats while limiting potential harm requires an awareness of safety factors and the establishment of dosage guidelines.

Toxicology and side effect risk are two of the main safety concerns when employing plant-based treatments for viral infections. Although bioactive molecules with therapeutic characteristics are present in medicinal plants, specific individuals may experience unpleasant reactions due to the presence of poisonous or allergic chemicals. For instance, pyrrolizidine alkaloids and ephedrine, which are found in herbs like comfrey and ephedra, can harm the liver and have an adverse effect on the circulatory system when taken in excess or over an extended period of time. Furthermore, some people may be allergic to specific herbs or plants, which can cause allergic reactions, including skin rashes, itching, or breathing symptoms. Therefore, in order to detect potential dangers and minimize them appropriately, it is imperative to analyze the safety profile of medicinal plants and natural chemicals through toxicological studies, pharmacovigilance monitoring, and clinical trials.

Another safety issue to keep in mind while using nature's pharmacy to treat viral threats is interactions between plant-based medicines and conventional pharmaceuticals. Certain botanical extracts and herbs can interact with pharmaceuticals, either increasing or decreasing their effects, which might result in adverse side effects or decreased effectiveness. For example, St. John's wort, a well-known herbal remedy for depression, may interfere with antiviral medications used to treat HIV/AIDS, such as protease inhibitors and non-nucleoside reverse transcriptase inhibitors, lowering drug levels and maybe even terminating treatment entirely. Similarly, anticoagulant drugs may interact with herbs like ginger, ginkgo biloba, and garlic, raising the risk of bleeding. Therefore, in order to prevent adverse effects when combining plant-based therapies with conventional pharmaceuticals, it is imperative to take into account potential herb-drug interactions and consult healthcare professionals.

Furthermore, defining dosage guidelines is crucial to guaranteeing the safety and effectiveness of plant-based treatments against viral threats. The right amount of natural substances and medicinal plants to use relies on a number of variables, including the type of plant, how it is prepared, the patient's age, weight, and overall health, as well as the desired therapeutic result. Dosage guidelines, which offer precise advice on dosage schedules, delivery methods, and treatment duration, aid in standardizing the use of plant-based medicines.

Dosage guidelines also consider the concentration and potency of bioactive substances found in herbal medicines, thereby reducing the risk of toxicity and ensuring that patients receive the correct therapeutic dose.

Furthermore, when determining dose guidelines for plant-based medicines, it is imperative to take into account the safety of sensitive populations, including pregnant women, children, and the elderly. For example, several herbs and botanical extracts may be advised against by pregnant women because of the possibility of negative effects on fetal development or pregnancy outcomes. Similar to adults, children may need fewer dosages of herbal treatments because of changes in metabolism and physiological responses, as well as smaller bodies. Furthermore, due to age-related changes in drug metabolism and clearance, older persons may be more vulnerable to drug interactions and side effects. To protect the safety and well-being of these populations, dosage recommendations should take into account their particular requirements and vulnerabilities.

Pharmacovigilance and risk management also depend on tracking and disclosing adverse events related to the use of plant-based treatments. Consumers, herbalists, and healthcare professionals should be encouraged to report any unanticipated results, adverse reactions, or side effects related to the use of herbal treatments in pharmacovigilance programs or regulatory bodies. Regulatory bodies can detect possible safety issues, put risk mitigation strategies in place, and revise dosage guidelines by methodically gathering and evaluating data on adverse events. Furthermore, encouraging open dialogue and transparency regarding the possible drawbacks and advantages of plant-based treatments encourages consumers and healthcare professionals to make responsible decisions and utilize them wisely.

In conclusion, using nature's pharmacy to effectively and safely combat viral threats requires careful consideration of safety concerns and dose requirements. Healthcare providers and patients can reduce the possibility of harm by using plant-based medicines wisely and by being aware of the possible risks, interactions, and side effects connected with them. The establishment of precise dosage standards guarantees standardized regimens and encourages dependability and consistency in the application of herbal treatments. Moreover, tracking and disclosing adverse events supports pharmacovigilance initiatives and helps protect the health and welfare of patients utilizing plant-based treatments for viral risks. The growing popularity of natural treatments has made it imperative to prioritize safety concerns and establish evidence-based dose guidelines in order to fully utilize nature's pharmacy in improving resilience against viral infections and overall health.

Creating Herbal Remedies at Home

Creating herbal remedies at home gives people an empowering and approachable way to tap into the healing power of plants in the search for natural ways to address viral threats. Herbal treatments manufactured from medicinal herbs and botanical extracts have been used for millennia in traditional medical systems all over the world because of their many therapeutic effects, which include antiviral activity. People can make a range of herbal remedies at home to strengthen their immune systems, relieve symptoms, and enhance general well-being by using basic techniques and readily accessible components. Homemade herbal treatments, which range from tinctures and teas to infused oils and salves, provide a holistic and natural way to combat viral threats while promoting sustainability, self-sufficiency, and a relationship with the natural world.

Herbal teas are among the most accessible and flexible herbal treatments you may make at home. Herbal teas are a soothing and satisfying beverage that are created by steeping fresh or dried medicinal herbs in hot water to release their health-promoting properties. Herbs with immune-boosting and antiviral qualities, such as elderberry, echinacea, ginger, lemon balm, and peppermint, are frequently used in herbal teas. For instance, elderberry tea has a high concentration of flavonoids and antioxidants that support immune system function and lessen the intensity and duration of viral infections. In a similar vein, ginger tea helps ease symptoms, including congestion, coughing, and sore throats, while echinacea tea is well-known for its immune-stimulating properties. Making herbal teas at home allows people to add natural protection against viral dangers while tailoring blends to their tastes and requirements.

Moreover, homemade herbal tinctures provide a concentrated and portable herbal medicine option, offering a tiny liquid form containing a solid dose of medicinal plant extracts. Medicinal plants are usually macerated in glycerin or alcohol to extract the active ingredients, which produces a concentrated liquid extract that can be consumed or mixed with drinks to make tinctures. Because of their antiviral, antibacterial, and immune-stimulating qualities, tinctures of herbs, including garlic, echinacea, oregano, and thyme, are frequently utilized. Allicin, a substance with potent antiviral properties, is present in garlic tincture, whereas echinacea tincture is abundant in immune-stimulating polysaccharides and alkylamides. Making herbal tinctures at home allows people to quickly adjust dosages and mixes to suit their particular needs while strengthening their defenses against viral illnesses.

Homemade herbal remedies can be applied topically to relieve symptoms and aid the body's natural healing processes in addition to being consumed. For instance, to extract the therapeutic components of dried or fresh herbs, olive, coconut, or jojoba oils are utilized as carriers when making herbal-infused oils. You can use infused oils as a base for DIY salves and balms or for massage and skin care applications. Because of their ability to reduce inflammation, act as an antibacterial, and aid in the healing of wounds, herbs including calendula, chamomile, lavender, plantain, and St. John's wort are frequently used in oils. For example, lavender-infused oil can help reduce stress, anxiety, and muscular tension; calendula-infused oil is helpful in easing skin irritations and encouraging wound healing. Making their own herbal-infused oils at home allows people to customize mixtures to target specific skin issues and improve general health.

Furthermore, applying herbal medicines topically for skin and respiratory conditions is made easy and portable with prepared herbal salves and balms. Beeswax or plant-based waxes are combined with herbal-infused oils to make salves, which are semi-solid ointments that are used topically for medicinal effects. Similar to salves, balms can also include extra components for extra nourishment and scent, including shea butter, cocoa butter, or essential oils. Because of their ability to assist the respiratory system and their antiviral and antibacterial qualities, herbs, including eucalyptus, peppermint, rosemary, tea tree, and thyme, are frequently used in salves and balms. For instance, you might apply eucalyptus salve to your chest or throat to ease congestion and encourage easier breathing.

Similarly, you can massage peppermint balm onto your temples and pulse points to ease headaches and encourage relaxation. Making herbal salves and balms at home allows people to practice self-care and self-sufficiency while producing customized natural treatments.

Additionally, including homemade herbal remedies in everyday routines might enhance general health and strengthen resistance to viral infections. For instance, fresh or dried herbs like thyme, peppermint, rosemary, or eucalyptus can be added to hot water and inhaled to open up the airways, reduce congestion, and support respiratory health. These herbs work well to relieve the symptoms of viral respiratory infections, including the flu, bronchitis, and colds. They include volatile oils that have antibacterial, expectorant, and decongestant qualities.

For instance, eucalyptus includes cineole, a substance with mucolytic and antiviral qualities, while peppermint has menthol, which eases congested airways and lessens coughing. People can improve their resistance to viral infections and boost respiratory health by including herbal steam inhalations in their regular routines.

To sum up, making herbal treatments at home gives people a flexible and empowering way to use plants' healing abilities to fend off viral threats. Handmade herbal remedies offer a variety of options for boosting immune system function, relieving symptoms, and enhancing general well-being, including tinctures, oils, and salves. People may create personalized herbal treatments that are suited to their unique health needs while promoting self-reliance, sustainability, and a connection with nature by using straightforward methods and widely available components. Homemade herbal treatments provide a natural and holistic way to manage viral threats while encouraging health, resilience, and well-being for everyone as interest in natural remedies continues to grow.

CHAPTER IX

Building Resilience with Plant-Based Antivirals

Lifestyle Practices to Support Immune Health

Adopting lifestyle choices that support immunological health is crucial to strengthening the body's defenses against viral threats and reducing the chance of infection. While advances in contemporary medicine offer valuable tools for fighting viral illnesses, a complementary and all-encompassing strategy for enhancing resilience against pathogens is to optimize immune function through lifestyle choices. Adopting behaviors that support general health can help people strengthen their immune systems, become less prone to infections, and be better able to fight off viral threats. Lifestyle choices, such as proper diet and hydration, stress reduction techniques, and sleep hygiene, are critical in promoting immune function and enhancing the body's natural defenses against viral infections.

Nutrition is one of the main pillars of immune health because the foods we eat offer us essential nutrients and antioxidants that boost immunological function. You can obtain a variety of vitamins, minerals, and phytonutrients that support immune system function and prevent disease by eating a diet high in fruits, vegetables, whole grains, lean meats, and healthy fats. The immune system depends on zinc, vitamin C, vitamin D, selenium, and zinc deficiency, all of which are linked to a higher risk of viral infections. To maintain the healthiest immune system and resistance to viral infections, a diet rich in nutrients and well-balanced is essential.

Furthermore, maintaining proper hydration is critical for promoting immune system performance and general wellness. Water is essential for several physiological functions, including as digestion, detoxification, and circulation, all of which support a robust immune system. It's important to stay hydrated throughout the day since dehydration can impair immune system performance and erode the body's resistance to infection. Herbal teas, broths, and fresh produce with a high water content, in addition to water, can help maintain hydration while offering extra nutrients and antioxidants that boost the function of the immune system. People can improve immune function and strengthen their defenses against viral threats by making drinking plenty of water a priority in their everyday routine.

Furthermore, keeping a robust and resilient immune system depends on giving adequate sleep a top priority. Immune function is largely regulated by sleep, with insufficient sleep being linked to weakened immune systems and greater vulnerability to infections. The body repairs and regenerates itself in several ways as we sleep, producing antibodies and cytokines to help fend off infections. Lack of sleep can also result in oxidative stress, inflammation, and deregulation of immunological pathways, all of which can impair immune function. Therefore, it is crucial to create good sleep hygiene practices to support immunological health and enhance resilience against viral threats. These activities include keeping a consistent sleep schedule, adopting a calming bedtime routine, and optimizing the sleep environment.

Effective stress management is also essential for maintaining immunological function and general well-being well being. Reducing immunological responses, increasing susceptibility to infections, and dysregulating the immune system are all consequences of chronic stress, so it's critical to learn stress-reduction strategies that foster resilience and relaxation. Techniques like tai chi, yoga, deep breathing, and mindfulness meditation can boost immunity, lower stress levels, and improve emotional health. Hobbies, time spent in nature, and relationships with loved ones can also build resilience against stressors and social support. People can boost their immune systems and lessen their susceptibility to viral threats by making stress management a daily priority.

In addition, regular exercise is essential for boosting immunity and strengthening resistance to illnesses. It has been shown that exercise improves circulation, reduces inflammation, and stimulates the production of immune cells—all of which contribute to a robust immune response. Frequent moderate-intensity physical activity, such riding a bike, swimming, or brisk walking, boosts immunity and reduces the risk of respiratory infections. In order to prevent immune suppression and overtraining, exercise needs to be tempered with adequate recovery time. People who engage in regular physical activity can improve their overall welfare, keep their immune systems strong, and fortify their defenses against viral threats.

Furthermore, avoiding the spread of pathogens and lowering the risk of viral infections requires adhering to strict cleanliness standards. Especially before eating or touching the face, frequent hand washing with soap and water can help remove bacteria and viruses from the skin and reduce the chance of transmission. Moreover, respiratory hygiene measures like covering the nostrils and mouth when coughing or sneezing, as well as avoiding direct contact with sick individuals, may aid in prevent the spread of respiratory viruses like influenza and coronaviruses. Furthermore, frequent cleaning and disinfection of high-touch areas including counters, doorknobs, and devices can help lower the risk of viral transmission at work and at home. People can reduce their chance of contracting viruses and safeguard others from disease by incorporating proper hygiene practices into their daily lives.

To sum up, lifestyle choices are critical for maintaining immunological function and enhancing the body's defense against viral infections. Making lifestyle choices that support general wellbeing—from eating and drinking right to managing stress and sleeping arrangements—improves immune system performance, lowers susceptibility to illnesses, and increases resistance to infections. People can enhance their immune systems and reduce their risk of viral infections by emphasizing a healthy diet, sufficient water, restful sleep, stress reduction, frequent exercise, and proper cleanliness. Investing in lifestyle habits that support immune health offers a proactive and comprehensive approach to promoting health and wellbeing for all, especially as the globe continues to confront persistent challenges from viral threats.

Incorporating Antiviral Foods and Herbs into Daily Routine

Including antiviral foods and herbs in daily routines provides a proactive, all-natural way to enhance immune health and lessen susceptibility to illnesses in the face of viral threats. Bioactive compounds that are present in antiviral foods and herbs have the capacity to impede the replication of viruses, fortify the immune system, and enhance the body's resistance against viral agents. By incorporating these powerful substances into regular meals, snacks, and drinks, people can leverage the medicinal properties of nature's pharmacy to fortify their resistance against infections. Adding antiviral foods and herbs into everyday routines is a quick and easy way to support general health and resilience against viral infections. These include immune-boosting fruits and vegetables as well as antimicrobial herbs and spices.

Stressing the importance of a diet high in immune-stimulating fruits and vegetables is one of the easiest methods to include antiviral foods in everyday activities. Rich in vitamins, minerals, antioxidants, and phytonutrients, fruits and vegetables are vital for boosting immune system performance and warding off illnesses. Citrus fruits with high vitamin C content include oranges, lemons, and grapefruits. Strong antioxidants like vitamin C aid in the development of white blood cells and antibodies, which are essential for warding off infections. Furthermore, the minerals zinc and selenium, along with the vitamins A, C, and E present in mysterious leafy greens like spinach, kale, and Swiss chard, fortify the body's defenses against viral infections. A person's body may get the nutrients it needs to keep its immune system strong and resilient by eating a variety of fruits and vegetables for breakfast, lunch, and snack throughout the day.

Additionally, adding taste and health benefits to meals through the everyday cooking of immune-boosting herbs and spices boosts immunity. Because they are antibacterial, anti-inflammatory, and immune-stimulating, herbs and spices like garlic, ginger, turmeric, oregano, and cinnamon are helpful additions to everyday cooking routines. For example, allicin, a component of garlic, possesses active antiviral and antibacterial properties that can help inhibit the growth of bacteria and viruses. Similarly, the anti-inflammatory and immune-boosting properties of gingerol and shogaol can help lessen the intensity and length of viral infections.

Additions of immune-boosting spices and herbs can boost the nutritional value of soups, stews, stir-fries, and other dishes while providing a natural barrier against viral invaders.

Moreover, adding antiviral foods and herbs to drinks like herbal teas, smoothies, and juices is a fun and easy method to maintain immune function all day long. Herbal teas with antiviral properties, derived from immune-stimulating herbs like peppermint, licorice root, echinacea, and elderberry, offer a calming and satisfying approach to staying hydrated. For instance, elderberry tea has a high concentration of flavonoids and antioxidants that support immune system function and lessen the intensity and duration of viral infections. In a similar vein, immune-supporting fruits and vegetables like spinach or kale, along with berries, kiwi, pineapple, and mango, can be blended into smoothies that are nutrient-rich and pleasant. Smoothies' antiviral qualities can be further enhanced by adding immune-boosting herbs and spices like cinnamon, ginger, and turmeric. Freshly squeezed juices from citrus fruits, apples, carrots, and ginger also create a vitamin-rich, hydrating drink that boosts immunity and has inherent antiviral properties. People may continuously protect their bodies against viral dangers while hydrating, nourishing, and fortifying them by adding antiviral foods and herbs to their beverages.

Additionally, adding antiviral foods and herbs to treats and snacks offers more ways to promote immune function while sating desires and increasing vitality. Trail mix, which consists of nuts, seeds, dried fruits, and dark chocolate, is a nutrient-dense, portable snack that boosts immunity and shields the body from free radical damage.

To further improve the nutritional content and antiviral qualities of homemade granola bars or energy balls, add immune-boosting herbs and spices like cayenne pepper, cinnamon, and turmeric. Additionally, making handmade sweets like energy bars, cookies, or bliss balls with immune-boosting components like raw honey, coconut oil, and bee pollen offers a tasty and nutritious snack choice. Through the use of antiviral foods and herbs in snacks and sweets, people can nourish their bodies with entire meals that boost immunity and enhance general health.

Moreover, integrating antiviral foods and herbs into regular meal preparation and cooking provides a proactive and long-term strategy to boost immune function and lessen vulnerability to viral infections. By giving immune-stimulating foods like fruits, vegetables, herbs, and spices priority, people may prepare tasty, nourishing meals that naturally guard against viral dangers. A quick and easy way to support immune function and resistance to infections is to incorporate antiviral foods and herbs into everyday routines. Some examples of these include adding garlic and ginger to stir- fries, turmeric, and cinnamon to smoothies, and elderberry and echinacea to herbal teas. Additionally, experimenting with new flavors and ingredients while broadening their repertoire of immune-boosting dishes is made possible by learning new recipes and culinary methods. People can proactively boost their immune systems and improve their capacity to fight viral threats by incorporating antiviral foods and herbs into their everyday cooking and meal planning.

Finally, adding antiviral foods and herbs to daily routines provides a proactive, all-natural way to boost immune function and lessen the risk of contracting viral illnesses. Integrating these powerful ingredients—which range from immune-boosting fruits and vegetables to antimicrobial herbs and spices—into meals, snacks, and drinks offers a quick and easy way to support general health and resilience against viral threats. Immune-boosting nutrients can be prioritized in everyday meal planning and cooking, allowing people to fuel their bodies with healthful foods that strengthen their defenses against illnesses. Incorporating antiviral foods and herbs into daily routines offers a proactive and empowering way to take responsibility for one's health and well-being as the globe continues to confront persistent difficulties from viral threats.

Empowering Individuals and Communities with Natural Solutions

Giving people and communities access to natural remedies in the face of viral threats is a proactive and long-term strategy for preventing infectious diseases. While modern medicine offers valuable resources for treating viral infections, utilizing nature's pharmacy offers a complementary and all-encompassing strategy for enhancing immune function and lowering susceptibility to infections. In addition to building resistance against viral risks, communities and individuals may take control of their health and wellbeing by encouraging information, access, and the incorporation of natural solutions into daily routines. Using natural remedies to empower individuals and communities offers a holistic approach to improving health, boosting immunity, and lessening the effects of viral infections. These remedies range from herbal cures and nutritional interventions to lifestyle changes and environmental measures.

In order to equip people and communities with sustainable responses to viral dangers, education is essential. People may make more educated decisions about their health and wellbeing when they are given accurate, evidence-based information about the advantages of natural medicines, foods that strengthen the immune system, and healthy lifestyle choices. Workshops, seminars, online materials, and community outreach programs are a few examples of educational projects that teach people how to incorporate natural remedies into their everyday routines. Through raising people's knowledge and awareness of the immune-boosting effects of diet, lifestyle choices, and herbs and supplements, education enables people to take preventative measures against viral illnesses, both in their communities and individually.

Having access to natural remedies is another crucial element in equipping people and communities to counteract viral threats successfully. People from a variety of socioeconomic situations can benefit from herbal treatments, dietary supplements, whole foods, and other natural interventions if these resources are made affordable and accessible. Access to locally grown, organic vegetables, medicinal herbs, and herbal treatments can be found at community gardens, farmers' markets, food cooperatives, and herbal dispensaries. These resources support self-sufficiency, sustainability, and good health. In addition, by offering instructional materials, incentives, and subsidies to marginalized groups, government policies, healthcare programs, and community-based efforts can facilitate access to natural solutions. Through the removal of obstacles to access and the encouragement of inclusivity, communities may enable people to take charge of their own health and wellbeing.

Incorporating natural remedies into everyday activities is crucial to equipping people and communities to proactively counteract viral threats. Educating people about the benefits of immune-boosting foods, herbal medicines, and healthy lifestyle choices can help them become more resilient to illnesses and enhance their general wellbeing. Initiatives like meal planning, cooking workshops, and recipe sharing can motivate people to make wholesome meals that boost immunity and offer organic defense against viral infections. Encouragement to utilize herbal teas, tinctures, and topical treatments for common conditions, including respiratory infections, the flu, and colds, also leads people to turn to nature's pharmacy for natural help. Incorporating stress-reduction strategies, physical activity regimens, and sleep hygiene practices into daily plans also assists people in making self-care and resilience-enhancing activities a priority. People can promote long-term health and immunity against viral dangers by incorporating natural treatments into everyday routines.

Furthermore, encouraging teamwork and collaboration between patients, medical experts, and neighborhood organizations bolsters attempts to counter viral dangers with non-toxic remedies. Communities can take advantage of a variety of resources and specialized knowledge by forming interdisciplinary teams and partnerships, which will enable them to design all-encompassing plans for enhancing health and wellbeing.

Natural solutions can be incorporated into clinical practice and patient care by healthcare professionals working in conjunction with herbalists, nutritionists, naturopaths, and other holistic practitioners. Together, community organizations, nonprofits, and grassroots projects can create educational efforts, disseminate materials, and push for laws that support natural approaches to wellness and health. Communities can use their collective knowledge, abilities, and resources to empower people and build resistance against viral threats by cultivating a culture of cooperation and teamwork.

Additionally, developing self-reliance and resilience at the individual and community levels is crucial to creating long-lasting solutions to counteract infectious threats. By encouraging resilience-building behaviors like flexibility, mindfulness, and community cohesion, people can acquire the abilities and assets needed to face obstacles head-on and triumph over adversity. Initiatives aimed at enhancing community resilience, such as mutual aid networks, community gardens, and disaster preparedness programs, facilitate the development of social ties, resourcefulness, and self-sufficiency while also promoting a feeling of group empowerment and unity and encouraging ecological resilience and lessening environmental stressors through sustainable living practices including organic farming, regenerative agriculture, and renewable energy benefits human health and wellbeing. Communities may lay the groundwork for long-term solutions to counter viral risks and advance everyone's health and wellbeing by encouraging resilience and self-reliance.

To sum up, equipping people and communities with natural remedies is a proactive and long-term strategy to counteract viral threats and advance resilience and health. Communities may empower individuals to take control of their health and wellbeing while developing resilience against infectious diseases by increasing information, access, and integration of natural therapies, foods, and lifestyle habits. In order to address viral threats with natural solutions, collaboration, cooperation, and resilience-building programs are strengthened. This lays the groundwork for long-term solutions that support everyone's health, wellbeing, and resilience. A route to a healthier, more resilient future is provided by arming people and communities with natural remedies as the globe continues to face challenges from viral dangers.

CHAPTER X

Modern Research and Discoveries

Advances in scientific understanding of plant-based antivirals

Scientists are looking more and more to nature's pharmacy for answers in the fight against viral threats, with a particular emphasis on the fantastic potential of plant-based antivirals. A wealth of bioactive chemicals with a variety of pharmacological characteristics, including intense antiviral action, can be found in the incredible biodiversity of plants. Scientific research throughout the years has advanced our knowledge of the mechanisms of action, safety profiles, and efficacy of plant-based antivirals, opening the door to their use as nature's response to viral threats. The scientific study of plant-based antivirals has promise for creating efficient and long-lasting treatments to fight a variety of viral infections, from conventional herbal therapies to cutting-edge drug discovery techniques.

Clarifying the molecular mechanisms of action of plant-based antivirals is one of the significant improvements in our understanding of these drugs. Numerous bioactive substances found in plants have been found by scientists to target different phases of the viral replication cycle and have antiviral effects. For instance, it has been demonstrated that polyphenols such as the epigallocatechin gallate (EGCG) present in green tea prevent the attachment and entry of viruses into host cells by obstructing viral binding sites or interfering with the processes involved in viral fusion. Similarly, alkaloids that are extracted from medicinal herbs like barberry and goldenseal, like berberine, show antiviral activity by preventing the replication of viruses or by blocking the enzymes that are necessary for the assembly and maturation of viruses. Scientists can create focused tactics to efficiently utilize plant-derived chemicals' antiviral potential by deciphering the complex interactions between these compounds and viral infections.

Furthermore, new antiviral agents from plant sources may now be precisely identified and characterized thanks to developments in phytochemistry and analytical methods. Extensive libraries of plant extracts can be screened by researchers using high-throughput screening assays, chromatography methods, and mass spectrometry analysis to identify bioactive chemicals with particular antiviral properties. By means of structural elucidation and bioassay-guided fractionation, researchers can pinpoint the chemical components that give rise to antiviral activity and enhance their effectiveness and potency. Moreover, the logical design of analogs and derivatives to improve antiviral activity, bioavailability, and safety profiles is made more accessible by computational methods and molecular modeling.

Through the application of contemporary analytical techniques, researchers can fully realize the antiviral potential of plant-based remedies in the fight against viral infections.

Furthermore, developments in pharmacology and pharmacokinetics have enhanced our comprehension of plant-based antivirals' safety and efficacy profiles in preclinical and clinical contexts. Preclinical research on in vitro and animal models offers essential insights into the pharmacokinetic characteristics, dose-response relationships, and antiviral mechanisms of drugs produced from plants. The pharmacodynamics and pharmacokinetics of plant-based antivirals, including their body's absorption, distribution, metabolism, and excretion, are clarified by pharmacological investigations. Clinical trials also assess the safety, tolerability, and effectiveness of plant-based antivirals in human subjects, offering fact-based information on their potential for therapeutic use and clinical value. Through a thorough evaluation of the pharmacological characteristics and safety profiles of antivirals derived from plants, researchers may create evidence-based guidelines for the prevention and treatment of viral infections.

Furthermore, our understanding of plant-based antivirals and their therapeutic applications has been enhanced by multidisciplinary approaches that combine traditional knowledge with contemporary scientific methodologies. Ethnobotanical research reveals how indigenous communities around the world have long used medicinal plants to treat a range of illnesses, including viral infections. By collaborating with indigenous communities and traditional healers, scientists can get valuable insights into the efficacy of conventional plant-based remedies in combating viral infections. Furthermore, phytochemical analysis and pharmacological research confirm the traditional applications of medicinal plants and pinpoint the active ingredients that give them their antiviral capabilities. Moreover, research on transcriptomics and genomes clarifies the molecular processes behind plant-virus interactions and the production of antiviral substances in plants. Through the integration of contemporary scientific methods with traditional knowledge, researchers can leverage the global collective wisdom of cultures to create innovative plant-based antivirals that are nature's response to viral threats.

Furthermore, the development of plant-based antivirals for therapeutic use has been transformed by breakthroughs in genetic engineering and biotechnology. Biotechnological techniques like tissue culture, plant cell culture, and metabolic engineering make it possible to produce bioactive chemicals in regulated settings on a large scale. Through genetic modification and culture optimization, researchers can increase the bioactivity, purity, and productivity of plant-derived antiviral chemicals. Furthermore, plant genomes can be modified to increase their resistance to viral infections or to increase the synthesis of bioactive compounds by genetic engineering techniques like gene editing and RNA interference. Furthermore, additional platforms for the synthesis of recombinant proteins and viral antigens for the development of vaccines and antiviral therapy are provided by plant-based expression systems, including bacteria, yeast, and plant viruses. Scientists can increase the therapeutic potential of plant-based antivirals and overcome resource availability constraints by utilizing genetic engineering techniques and biotechnological technologies.

Plant-based antivirals have also been made more accessible for formulation and administration for improved efficacy and targeted administration thanks to developments in nanotechnology and drug delivery systems. For plant-derived chemicals, nanoparticle-based formulations such as liposomes, polymeric nanoparticles, and lipid nanoparticles provide benefits like enhanced tissue targeting, stability, and bioavailability. Scientists are able to preserve bioactive substances from deterioration, increase their solubility, and extend the duration of their bodily circulation by encasing them in nanoparticles. Furthermore, the ability to functionalize nanoparticles with targeting ligands facilitates the targeted delivery of antiviral agents to certain viral pathogen-infected cells or tissues. Moreover, nanotechnology-based techniques make the co-delivery of several bioactive chemicals or synergistic combinations of synthetic and plant-derived antivirals for increased efficacy against viral infections possible. Scientists can overcome obstacles to the clinical translation of plant-based antivirals and maximize their therapeutic effects for nature's response to viral threats by utilizing nanotechnology and drug delivery systems.

In conclusion, the search for and application of plant-based antivirals as nature's response to viral threats has been accelerated by breakthroughs in scientific understanding. Scientists have made significant progress in unlocking the therapeutic potential of plant-based antivirals, from clarifying their mechanisms of action to identifying novel bioactive compounds, optimizing their efficacy and safety profiles, fusing traditional knowledge with contemporary scientific methodologies, utilizing genetic engineering and biotechnological approaches, and utilizing nanotechnology and drug delivery systems. Scientists can battle a broad spectrum of viral diseases with sustainable and effective remedies by collaborating across disciplines and continuing to innovate. This will pave the path for a more robust and healthy future for everybody.

Case studies of plant compounds with proven antiviral activity

Researchers have looked to nature's pharmacopeia to investigate the potential of plant chemicals as antiviral medicines in the ongoing fight against viral threats. Numerous plant chemicals with demonstrated antiviral action have surfaced via thorough scientific research, providing encouraging treatments for a range of viral diseases. These case studies shed light on the mechanisms of action, efficacy, and possible therapeutic applications of the wide range of plant-based substances that possess antiviral solid characteristics.

A prominent example of a case study is the flavonoid component quercetin, which is present in large quantities in a wide range of fruits, vegetables, and medicinal plants. The antiviral activity of quercetin against a variety of viruses, including influenza, herpes simplex virus, respiratory syncytial virus, and coronaviruses, has been the subject of much research. According to research, quercetin works against viruses by reducing their ability to replicate, preventing their adhesion to and penetration into host cells, and adjusting the immune system of the host. Additionally, quercetin has anti-inflammatory and antioxidant qualities, which may help it lessen tissue damage and inflammation brought on by viruses. Quercetin has shown promise in lowering the intensity and duration of viral infections in clinical investigations, suggesting that it is a good candidate for further research as a natural antiviral medication.

Polyphenol resveratrol, which is present in berries, red wine, peanuts, and grapes, is the subject of another interesting case study. Resveratrol has garnered attention because of its wide-range protective properties against a range of viruses, including coronaviruses, hepatitis C virus (HCV), influenza, and human immunodeficiency virus (HIV). Resveratrol enhances antiviral defense systems by suppressing viral gene expression, inhibiting viral replication, and modulating host immunological responses, according to studies. Furthermore, resveratrol has immunomodulatory, anti-inflammatory, and antioxidant properties, which may help explain how well it fights viral infections. Resveratrol's promise as a natural antiviral medication has been highlighted by clinical trials that show it is effective in lowering viral load, improving clinical outcomes, and boosting immune function in patients with viral infections.

In addition, curcumin—a polyphenol obtained from the turmeric plant—has shown promise as a solid antiviral drug with broad-spectrum efficacy against a range of viruses, such as the dengue virus, herpes simplex virus, influenza, and human papillomavirus (HPV). In order to strengthen antiviral defense mechanisms, curcumin modulates host immunological responses, prevents viral replication, and interferes with the creation of viral proteins. In addition, curcumin has immunomodulatory, anti-inflammatory, and antioxidant qualities that may help it fight viral infections. Curcumin has shown promise as a natural antiviral medication in clinical trials by effectively lowering viral load and symptomatic and improving clinical outcomes in individuals with viral infections.

Furthermore, berberine, an alkaloid present in a variety of medicinal plants including Oregon grape, barberry, and goldenseal, has demonstrated encouraging antiviral activity against a variety of viruses, including respiratory syncytial virus, herpes simplex virus, influenza, and human cytomegalovirus (HCMV). By targeting viral enzymes and interfering with viral DNA synthesis or RNA transcription, berberine prevents the spread of viruses.

Additionally, berberine has immunomodulatory properties that strengthen the host immune system's ability to fight viral infections. Berberine's promise as a natural antiviral medication has been highlighted by clinical trials that show it is effective in lowering viral load, improving clinical outcomes, and boosting immune function in patients with viral infections.

Additionally, green tea catechin called epigallocatechin gallate (EGCG) has shown potent antiviral properties against a number of viruses, such as influenza, hepatitis B virus (HBV), human herpesvirus (HHV), and human papillomavirus (HPV). By targeting viral enzymes and obstructing the production of viral DNA or RNA, EGCG prevents the spread of viruses. In addition, EGCG has immunomodulatory, anti-inflammatory, and antioxidant qualities that may help it fight viral infections. Research on individuals with viral infections has demonstrated that EGCG can lower viral load, relieve symptoms, and improve clinical outcomes; these findings raise the possibility of EGCG being used as a natural antiviral treatment.

In summary, these case studies highlight the diverse range of plant compounds that exhibit antiviral characteristics, offering promising strategies for mitigating viral risks. These plant-derived substances, which include flavonoids like quercetin, polyphenols like resveratrol, curcumin, and EGCG, and alkaloids like berberine, have strong antiviral properties against a range of viruses. Numerous studies conducted in preclinical and clinical settings have examined their modes of action, effectiveness, and safety profiles, highlighting their promise as natural antiviral treatments. Researchers can create sustainable and effective solutions for nature's response to viral threats by utilizing the medicinal potential of these plant chemicals, providing promise for a healthier and more resilient future.

CHAPTER XI

Integrative Approaches to Viral Prevention and Treatment

Combining plant-based antivirals with conventional therapies

Researchers are delving deeper into the possibility of integrating plant-based antivirals with traditional treatments in the fight against viral threats in order to create more potent and all-encompassing therapeutic approaches. Conventional antiviral medications are essential for treating viral infections, but they frequently have drawbacks such as narrow-spectrum action, side effects, and drug resistance. When used with traditional medicines, plant-based antivirals may have synergistic effects due to their various modes of action, reduced side effects, and prospective alternatives. Through the use of the complementing characteristics of both conventional and plant-based antivirals, scientists hope to improve treatment outcomes, combat medication resistance, and lessen the prevalence of viral infections worldwide.

To increase efficacy and lower the potential of medication resistance, one strategy for combining plant-based antivirals with conventional medicines is to target distinct stages of the viral replication cycle. Plant-based antivirals may work through different mechanisms, such as blocking viral attachment and entry, modifying host immune responses, or directly causing virucidal effects. Conventional antiviral medications usually target specific viral enzymes or proteins involved in viral replication. Researchers can establish synergistic interactions that increase antiviral efficacy and decrease the chance of viral resistance evolving by combining drugs that target various points in the viral replication cycle. Combining a protease inhibitor, for instance, with a plant-derived substance that targets viral attachment or fusion may boost overall antiviral efficacy and stop the emergence of viral escape variants.

Furthermore, integrating plant-based antivirals with traditional treatments can enhance patient results and lessen the negative consequences of long-term conventional medication use. The gastrointestinal problems, hepatotoxicity, and nephrotoxicity that are frequent side effects of conventional antiviral medications can make them less tolerable and reduce treatment compliance. Conversely, plant-based antivirals are appealing options for combination therapy since they are typically well-tolerated and have fewer side effects.

Researchers can minimize adverse effects while maintaining therapeutic efficacy by reducing the dosage and duration of conventional medications by adding plant-based antivirals into therapy regimens. Furthermore, plant-based chemicals' anti-inflammatory, immunomodulatory, and antioxidant qualities may lessen tissue damage and inflammation brought on by viral infections, enhancing patient outcomes and quality of life even more.

Additionally, the issue of drug resistance, which continues to be a major concern in the field of antiviral therapy, can be addressed by combining plant-based antivirals with conventional medicines. Viral pathogens can remarkably evolve resistance to conventional treatments by selecting drug-resistant variants or causing changes in their genomes. Combination therapy, which combines plant-based antivirals with conventional medications, can target several viral proteins or host cell components involved in the viral replication cycle, thereby improving treatment outcomes and lowering the risk of drug resistance developing. Furthermore, plant-based chemicals might be effective against a variety of viral strains or kinds across a broad spectrum, which makes them a useful addition to traditional treatments for infections that are resistant to drugs. Researchers can create more resilient and long-lasting treatment plans that can handle the difficulties of drug resistance and guarantee long-term efficacy in treating viral infections by combining drugs with complementary mechanisms of action.

Additionally, combining plant-based antivirals with traditional treatments can boost the effectiveness of antivirals and improve the course of treatment for viral infections that are developing or re-emerging. Novel viral infections like SARS-CoV-2, the Zika virus, and the Ebola virus have emerged in recent years and represent serious threats to the security of global health. The need for alternate treatment options is highlighted by the possibility that conventional antiviral medications will not be as effective against these developing viruses. Plant-based antivirals are appealing candidates for combination therapy because they provide a wide range of bioactive chemicals with broad-spectrum activity against several viral infections. Researchers can create more potent and flexible treatment regimens that can successfully restrict the spread of new viral infections and lessen their impact on public health by mixing plant-based antivirals with conventional medications.

Additionally, especially in areas with limited resources, combining plant-based antivirals with conventional medicines can help resolve discrepancies in access to antiviral treatment. Because of their high cost, many people in low- and middle-income countries—where the burden of viral infections is disproportionately large—are unable to afford conventional antiviral medications. Plant-based antivirals are readily grown, processed, and given to underprivileged areas as an inexpensive, sustainable, and locally accessible option. Researchers can lessen healthcare delivery gaps and increase access to effective antiviral medicines by incorporating plant-based antivirals into current healthcare systems and treatment methods. Additionally, local communities can be empowered to take charge of their health and well-being and harness the healing power of nature through the use of herbal medicine gardens, community-based projects, and traditional medical practices.

To sum up, integrating plant-based antivirals with traditional treatments presents a viable strategy for thwarting viral threats and enhancing global health outcomes. Combination therapy, which involves using conventional drugs and plant-based antivirals to target different stages of the viral replication cycle, has the potential to be nature's solution to viral threats. It can also overcome drug resistance, mitigate side effects, improve treatment accessibility, and increase the efficacy of antiviral treatments. As this field of study develops, scientists will need to work across disciplines and take advantage of the synergistic interactions between conventional and plant-based therapies to create novel treatment approaches that will effectively control viral infections and advance everyone's health and well-being.

Role of nutrition and lifestyle in supporting immune function

Diet and lifestyle choices are crucial to maintaining immunological function and strengthening the body's defenses against viral assaults. A robust immune system is maintained by a variety of lifestyle factors, including stress management, regular physical activity, a well- balanced diet high in nutrients, and enough sleep. Optimizing diet and lifestyle choices becomes even more critical when it comes to viral infections because they have a direct impact on the body's capacity to develop a protective immune response, ward off pathogens, and lessen the severity of infections. Gaining an understanding of the complex interactions among immune function, lifestyle, and diet is crucial to utilizing nature's defense against viral threats and enhancing general health and well-being well being.

Diet plays a vital role in regulating immunological response and bolstering the body's defenses against viral infections. Vital nutrients for immune cell activity, antioxidant protection, and immunological control include zinc, selenium, vitamins A, C, D, and E, and omega-3 fatty acids. For instance, vitamin D controls immune cell activity and influences inflammatory responses, whereas vitamin C promotes the development of immune cells, including phagocytes and lymphocytes. Zinc aids in the development and operation of immune cells, while selenium serves as an antioxidant and enhances immune cell performance. Eating a wide variety of complete meals that include lean proteins, whole grains, nuts, seeds, and fruits and vegetables guarantees that these vital nutrients are adequately ingested and supports a strong immune system.

Furthermore, plant-based diets contain phytochemicals that have immunomodulatory solid qualities and support the body's fight against viral infections. Antioxidant, anti-inflammatory, and antiviral properties of phytochemicals such as flavonoids, polyphenols, carotenoids, and glucosinolates boost immune system performance and lower the risk of viral infections. For instance, studies have demonstrated that flavonoids, which are present in berries, citrus fruits, and green tea, improve immune cell performance and prevent the spread of viruses. In a similar vein, polyphenols found in herbs like garlic and spices like turmeric have antiviral qualities that support a healthy immune system. People can enhance their body's natural defenses against viral threats and benefit from the immune-boosting properties of phytochemicals by including a diverse range of plant-based foods in their diet.

Moreover, immune system optimization and viral infection susceptibility reduction depend on leading a healthy lifestyle. Frequent exercise has been demonstrated to boost circulation, strengthen immunological surveillance, and enhance general health. Exercise lowers inflammation, boosts the body's defenses against infections, and stimulates the development of immune cells. Furthermore, as sleep deprivation can compromise immune function and heighten susceptibility to infections, getting enough sleep is crucial for maintaining immunological health. Antibody responses, cytokine synthesis, and immune cell proliferation are all aided by sleep and are necessary for creating a potent defense against viral infections.

Another crucial component of boosting immunity and lessening the effects of viral risks is stress management. It has been demonstrated that long-term stress reduces inflammation, impairs immunological function, and makes people more susceptible to infections. Deep breathing exercises, yoga, mindfulness meditation, and relaxation techniques are some examples of stress-reduction practices that can help reduce stress hormones, boost immunity, and increase resistance to viral infections. In addition, keeping a healthy weight, abstaining from tobacco use, consuming little alcohol, and adopting proper hygiene practices like handwashing and respiratory etiquette is critical for lowering the risk of viral infections and enhancing general health.

Environmental factors are essential in promoting immune function and reducing viral risks, in addition to dietary and lifestyle factors. Sunlight exposure is necessary for the manufacture of vitamin D, which is essential for immune regulation and antiviral defense. Immune system support and appropriate vitamin D levels can be maintained by spending time outside, participating in outdoor activities, and receiving enough sunlight. Reducing exposure to pollutants, poisons, and infectious agents in the environment can also lessen the strain on the immune system and help prevent viral infections. To sustain immune function and defend against viral assaults, a clean environment, clean air, and clean water are necessary.

In addition, the gut microbiota is essential for immunological control and viral infection prevention. The generation of antimicrobial peptides, immune system support, and gut barrier integrity are all bolstered by a varied and well-balanced gut microbiota. Having a diet high in fiber, probiotics, and prebiotics nourishes the good bacteria in the stomach and supports the health of the microbiome. Probiotic-rich foods including kefir, sauerkraut, kimchi, and yogurt help maintain a healthy gut flora and function of the immune system. Probiotic-rich foods, including yogurt, kefir, sauerkraut, and kimchi, help maintain gut health and immune system function. Through nutrition and lifestyle decisions, people can support a healthy gut microbiome, boost immunity, and lower their risk of viral infections.

To sum up, diet and lifestyle are crucial for maintaining immune system health and strengthening the body's defenses against viral invaders. Strong immunity is a result of a variety of factors, including environmental influences, stress management, regular exercise, a well-balanced diet high in nutrients, and enough sleep. People can enhance their immune systems and lessen their vulnerability to viral infections by including foods that strengthen the immune system, adopting healthy lifestyle habits, and limiting their exposure to environmental pollutants. A comprehensive strategy for boosting immune function and encouraging nature's defense against viral threats is to take advantage of the synergistic effects of diet, lifestyle, and environmental variables. As this field of study develops, strengthening resistance to viral infections and improving general health and wellbeing will depend on providing communities and individuals with the information and tools they need to adopt healthy practices.

Holistic approaches to viral prevention and management

Adopting holistic approaches to the management and prevention of viral risks provides a comprehensive strategy that supports the body's natural defenses against infections and utilizes resources found in nature. In order to effectively prevent and control viral infections, holistic healthcare recognizes the interconnectedness of mind, body, and spirit and emphasizes the need to correct underlying imbalances and foster general well-being. Holistic approaches provide nature's solution to viral dangers beyond conventional medical interventions by combining various modalities such as herbal therapy, mind-body practices, environmental concerns, lifestyle modifications, and diet.

In order to maintain immune function and guard against viral infections, nutrition is essential. Whole foods, fruits, vegetables, lean meats, healthy fats, and complex carbohydrates are good sources of nutrients that are high in vitamins, minerals, antioxidants, and phytochemicals that boost immunity and lessen the risk of infection. The body's natural defenses against viral threats can be strengthened by including immune-boosting foods like citrus fruits, berries, leafy greens, garlic, ginger, turmeric, and medicinal mushrooms in the diet. In addition, abstaining from processed meals, sugar-filled drinks, and heavy alcohol use supports gut health, lowers inflammation, and enhances immune system performance.

In apart from reducing the probability of infection from viruses, leading a healthy lifestyle also improves overall health and wellbeing. Maintaining a healthy immune system and stopping the spread of viruses requires handwashing, respiratory etiquette, environmental cleanliness, stress management, and frequent physical activity. Adequate sleep promotes immune cell activity, cytokine synthesis, and antibody responses, whereas exercise increases immune surveillance, decreases inflammation, and improves circulation. Deep breathing exercises, yoga, mindfulness meditation, and relaxation techniques are some of the stress-reduction strategies that can help reduce stress hormones, strengthen the immune system, and increase resistance to illnesses.

Vital antiviral natural ingredients found in herbal medicine can boost immune system performance and lessen viral infections. For millennia, people have utilized herbal treatments made from plants, including echinacea, elderberry, licorice root, astragalus, Andrographis, and olive leaf extract, to prevent and treat viral infections. These plants include bioactive substances with antiviral, anti-inflammatory, and immunomodulatory properties, including flavonoids, polyphenols, alkaloids, terpenoids, and polysaccharides. Herbal treatments can strengthen the body's defenses against viral threats and hasten the healing process from infections when added to holistic therapy methods.

Mind-body therapies, including yoga, tai chi, qigong, meditation, and acupuncture, provide comprehensive methods for boosting immunity, lowering stress levels, and improving general well-being. In order to maximize health and strengthen resistance to infections, these age-old therapeutic modalities concentrate on reestablishing harmony and balance within the body, mind, and spirit. While yoga and tai chi encourage relaxation, flexibility, and circulation, meditation and mindfulness techniques assist in quieting the mind, reducing stress, and controlling immunological reactions. The body's energy pathways are stimulated, yin and yang energies are balanced, and the body's defenses against infections are reinforced by acupuncture and traditional Chinese medicine treatments.

Since the environment has a significant impact on immune function and susceptibility to infections, environmental factors are crucial in comprehensive approaches to viral prevention and management. Clean water, air, and surroundings strengthen the immune system and reduce the risk of virus transmission.

Reducing the immune system's workload and preventing viral infections can be achieved by minimizing exposure to poisons, pollutants, and infectious agents in the environment. Furthermore, engaging in outdoor activities, fostering a sense of environmental responsibility, and spending time in nature all contribute to general well-being and resistance to viral risks.

Moreover, community-based strategies for managing and preventing viral infections are essential parts of comprehensive medical care. Giving people and communities access to information, tools, and support systems increases communal immunity to viral infections and promotes collective resilience. Collaborative efforts among stakeholders are encouraged, healthy behaviors are promoted, and effective prevention techniques are brought to light through educational initiatives, public health campaigns, and community outreach programs. In the face of infectious risks, community-based initiatives improve individual and communal wellbeing by creating a supportive atmosphere that fosters solidarity, cooperation, and shared responsibility.

To sum up, holistic methods of managing and preventing viral infections combine lifestyle modifications, herbal remedies, mind-body techniques, community-based strategies, environmental factors, and nutrition to provide nature's solution to viral dangers. Holistic medicine addresses the relationship between the mind, body, spirit, and environment and helps people become resilient and immune to viral diseases. Adopting holistic values enables people to take charge of their health, develop resilience, and confidently and powerfully negotiate the complexity of viral dangers. In the face of numerous problems, nature's wisdom offers an enduring roadmap for improving health, harmony, and vitality as science and our understanding of holistic approaches grow.

CHAPTER XII

Future Directions and Challenges

Emerging trends in plant-based antiviral research
Growing interest has been shown in plant-based antivirals as viable substitutes against viral dangers, providing safe, long-term remedies for viral illnesses. A number of new developments in this field of study are reshaping the field of plant-based antiviral research and spurring creativity and ingenuity in the search for a natural remedy for viral threats. These trends offer exciting opportunities to harness the therapeutic potential of plants in the fight against viral infections. Novel plant sources, bioactive component identification, synergistic combinations, sustainable extraction techniques, and therapeutic applications are just a few of the many topics they cover.

Investigating novel plant sources and conventional medical systems to find new bioactive chemicals with strong antiviral effects is a popular approach in plant-based antiviral research. To find hidden gems in nature's pharmacy, researchers are increasingly relying on ethnobotanical expertise and ancient medical practices. Indigenous plants have a vast biological diversity and cultural legacy, making them a valuable source of medicinal plants with unrealized antiviral potential. These plants are used in ancient medical systems, including Ayurveda, ancient Chinese Medicine, and Indigenous healing practices. Researchers can find novel antiviral medicines and confirm their effectiveness through scientific validation by methodically screening plant extracts and bioactive components produced from traditional medicinal plants.

Furthermore, new developments in computer modeling, high-throughput screening techniques, and analytical methodologies have entirely changed the way bioactive chemicals derived from plants are identified and characterized. Nuclear magnetic resonance (NMR) spectroscopy, bioinformatics, and liquid chromatography- mass spectrometry (LC-MS) are a few techniques that scientists use to precisely separate bioactive compounds and analyze the chemical composition of plant extracts. Moreover, the prediction of putative antiviral drugs and their modes of action is made easier by virtual screening, molecular docking, and structure-activity relationship (SAR) investigations, which speed up drug discovery efforts and direct logical drug design techniques.

Another new development in the field is the mechanistic understanding of plant-based drugs' antiviral activity, which offers important insights into their mode of action and therapeutic potential. Scientists are dissecting the molecular processes that underlie plant chemicals' antiviral activity and clarifying how these interact with immune signaling pathways, host cell components, and viral targets. For example, studies have shown that certain flavonoids target viral enzymes to stop the spread of viruses or limit the entry of viruses into host cells.

Furthermore, polyphenols have immunomodulatory properties that strengthen the host immune system's ability to fight viral infections. Researchers can maximize the therapeutic efficiency of plant chemicals and provide targeted therapies for certain viral illnesses by understanding the complex interactions that occur between these compounds and viral pathogens.

A promising tactic to improve antiviral efficacy and combat drug resistance is the synergistic combining of plant-based antivirals with conventional medications or other plant chemicals. In order to optimize antiviral activity, researchers are investigating synergistic interactions between plant components and utilizing the complementary qualities of various bioactive chemicals. Combining flavonoids with alkaloids or polyphenols, for instance, may enhance their antiviral properties by influencing complementary antiviral pathways or focusing on different stages of the viral replication cycle. Additionally, drug resistance can be defeated, and treatment outcomes against resistant viral strains can be improved by combining plant-based antivirals in synergistic combinations with conventional medications. Researchers can create more potent and long-lasting antiviral treatments for viruses by utilizing the synergistic relationships among plant components. This is nature's response to viral threats.

The use of green technology and sustainable extraction techniques is becoming more common in plant-based antiviral research, a reflection of the public's rising concern for environmental preservation and moral issues in medicine development. Modern extraction techniques, including supercritical fluid extraction (SFE), ultrasound-assisted extraction (UAE), and microwave-assisted extraction (MAE), are being used in addition to traditional procedures like maceration, decoction, and infusion.

These environmentally friendly technologies include benefits like lower solvent use, faster extraction times, greater extraction yields, and integrity preservation of bioactive components. Additionally, socially and ecologically responsible supply chains are ensured by sustainable sourcing techniques, organic farming methods, and fair-trade programs, all of which support the preservation of cultural traditions, socioeconomic growth, and biodiversity in communities that use medicinal plants.

Plant-based antivirals are showing their safety, effectiveness, and therapeutic potential in treating viral infections as they move from preclinical research to human trials. The efficacy of plant-based antivirals against certain viral illnesses, such as influenza, herpes simplex virus, human immunodeficiency virus, and coronaviruses, is presently being investigated through clinical trials. These trials will yield important information regarding the clinical utility and dose regimens of these drugs. Additionally, to maximize treatment outcomes and enhance patient care, integrative strategies that incorporate plant-based antivirals with conventional treatments, immunomodulators, or supportive care measures are being investigated. Researchers can confirm the effectiveness of plant-based antivirals and open the door for their incorporation into traditional healthcare systems by bringing preclinical research into clinical practice.

In summary, new directions in plant-based antiviral research are propelling creativity and learning in the hunt for a natural defense against viral infections. Researchers are effectively using plants' therapeutic potential to fight viral infections through a variety of approaches, including investigating new plant sources, identifying bioactive compounds, clarifying their mechanisms of action, utilizing combinations that work well together, implementing sustainable extraction techniques, and advancing clinical applications. Plant-based antivirals offer promising options for regulating viral risks and boosting global health and well-being because they prioritize ethical and environmental concerns, embrace interdisciplinary cooperation, and integrate traditional knowledge with modern scientific approaches. Nature's Pharmacy offers countless chances to treat the problems caused by viral infections and promote a healthier and more resilient future for all as long as research in this area continues to advance.

Regulatory issues and commercialization challenges

Numerous regulatory and commercialization obstacles stand in the way of the development and widespread use of natural products, such as plant-based antivirals, to combat viral threats. While plant-based remedies seem like nature's solution to viral threats, researchers, manufacturers, and entrepreneurs face many challenges in navigating regulatory frameworks, guaranteeing product quality and safety, protecting intellectual property rights, breaking through market barriers, and addressing ethical issues.

A significant regulatory obstacle in the creation of plant-based antivirals is the intricate and frequently strict regulatory environments controlling the authorization, production, and distribution of herbal remedies. Significant preclinical and clinical data are needed by regulatory agencies such as the FDA, which stands for the Food and Drug Administration, the European Medicines Agency (EMA), along with additional national regulatory authorities to demonstrate safety, efficacy, and quality criteria for drug approval. However, compared to synthetic pharmaceuticals, traditional herbal medicines frequently need more standardized formulations, constant potency, and rigorous clinical data, making it difficult to comply with regulatory regulations.

Furthermore, different countries classify plant-based products differently as dietary supplements, herbal remedies, or traditional medicines, which further complicates the regulatory environment and raises questions about their commercialization.

The commercialization of plant-based antivirals is hampered by the enormous hurdles of guaranteeing product quality, safety, and consistency. Variations in plant species, growth circumstances, harvesting practices, extraction procedures, and formulation techniques might lead to uneven potency, purity, and bioavailability of the final product. Pesticide, heavy metal, microbial pathogen, or adulterant contamination exacerbates safety worries and problems with regulatory compliance. Good manufacturing practices (GMP), quality control techniques, and standard testing protocols must be implemented in order to achieve product quality and safety throughout the production process. However, small-scale producers and practitioners of traditional medicine may need help to enter the market due to the increased expenses, infrastructure, and technical skills that these steps imply.

Another obstacle to plant-based antiviral commercialization is securing intellectual property rights. Because of their inherent unpredictability and broad usage in traditional medicine, natural medications produced from plants are frequently subject to limited patent protection, in contrast to synthetic drugs, which can be patented based on innovative chemical structures or manufacturing processes. It can be challenging to prove uniqueness, ingenuity, and utility when trying to patent bioactive chemicals, extraction processes, formulation techniques, or particular uses of plant-based antivirals because of prior art and body of knowledge in the industry. Furthermore, the commercialization of plant-based medicines frequently incorporates customs and knowledge from indigenous cultures, creating moral and legal questions around benefit-sharing, intellectual property rights, and the preservation of cultural heritage.

Significant commercialization problems for plant-based antivirals include breaking through market obstacles and winning over consumers. Synthetic medications with well-defined chemical structures, dependable pharmacokinetics, and established regulatory processes for market approval are often preferred by the pharmaceutical industry. Because of the perceived efficacy, safety, and standardization issues, natural products—including plant-based remedies—frequently encounter skepticism, regulatory scrutiny, and obstacles to market entry. Furthermore, market penetration and patient access to plant-based antivirals are further restricted by the absence of funding systems, insurance coverage, and approval from healthcare providers. In order to overcome these obstacles to the market, industry players, government organizations, medical professionals, and legislators must work together to create a climate of confidence, provide data, and create channels for the sale of plant-based antivirals.

The commercialization of plant-based antivirals raises ethical questions of cultural appropriation, biopiracy, indigenous rights, and equitable benefit distribution. Indigenous people have long utilized a variety of endemic plant species with medicinal qualities for healing and well-being. Without sufficient consent, benefit-sharing agreements, or respect for indigenous rights, the commercial exploitation of traditional medicinal knowledge, genetic resources, and biodiversity poses ethical questions and runs the risk of perpetuating historical injustices. To ensure the ethical and socially acceptable commercialization of plant-based antivirals, it is imperative to engage with indigenous stakeholders, respect traditional knowledge systems, stimulate community involvement, and follow fair trade procedures.

In conclusion, there are significant obstacles to the development and market access of plant-based antivirals for combating viral threats, including regulatory concerns and commercialization difficulties. Collaboration among researchers, manufacturers, lawmakers, and community stakeholders is essential to address ethical dilemmas, surmount market barriers, safeguard intellectual property rights, negotiate intricate regulatory environments, and guarantee product safety and quality. To fully utilize nature's power to address viral risks and advance global health and well-being, collaborative approaches that incorporate traditional knowledge, scientific innovation, regulatory expertise, and ethical considerations are needed. Plant-based antivirals have great potential as nature's response to viral threats, and their full realization will depend on creating an enabling environment that strikes a balance between innovation, regulation, and ethical stewardship as research and commercialization initiatives advance.

Potential impact of plant-based antivirals on global health

Plant-based antivirals have a wide range of potential effects on global health and present new ways to combat the rising threat of viral infections in the world. Plant-based antivirals provide the potential to transform the field of viral prevention, management, and therapy due to their wide range of bioactive chemicals, broad- spectrum effectiveness against viral infections, sustainable sourcing methods, and cultural significance. Plant-based antivirals have the potential to improve global health outcomes, strengthen resistance to viral threats, and provide fair access to effective antiviral medicines for all people by utilizing nature's pharmacy.

The ability of plant-based antivirals to increase the treatment options available for treating viral infections is one of their main potential effects on global health, especially in resource-constrained situations where access to traditional antiviral medications is frequently restricted. Numerous plant species possessing antiviral qualities are native to areas where viral diseases like dengue fever, malaria, Zika virus, and respiratory infections are highly prevalent. Native American-based traditional medical systems have long used plant-based treatments to prevent and treat viral infections. These treatments provide accessible, reasonably priced, and culturally appropriate substitutes for pharmaceuticals.

Researchers can increase access to efficient antiviral medicines, lessen healthcare inequities, and improve health outcomes in marginalized groups by incorporating plant-based antivirals into conventional healthcare systems and treatment protocols.

Furthermore, the potential benefits of plant-based antivirals go beyond their ability to treat illness; they also include more comprehensive benefits to public health, environmental sustainability, and socioeconomic advancement. Plant-based medicines are frequently grown, collected, and processed utilizing conventional and environmentally friendly techniques that support ecosystem resilience, biodiversity preservation, and environmental stewardship. In addition to helping local economies and rural communities, researchers and manufacturers can protect traditional knowledge and medicinal plant resources for future generations by promoting fair-trade programs, organic farming techniques, and sustainable sourcing practices. In addition, the incorporation of plant-based antivirals into public health campaigns, community-based programs, and primary healthcare systems can enable people to take charge of their health, encourage preventive actions, and lessen the spread of viral diseases.

The ability of plant-based antivirals to battle new and re-emerging viral diseases that endanger the security of global health is another meaningful potential impact on global health. The emergence of new viral epidemics, including avian influenza, Zika virus, Ebola virus, and SARS-CoV-2, highlights the critical need for creative antiviral tactics that can stop the spread of illnesses and lessen their adverse effects on public health. Plant-based antivirals are valuable tools in the battle against newly developing viral threats because they provide a wide range of bioactive chemicals with broad-spectrum activity against various viral strains and kinds. Researchers are able to create flexible antiviral treatments that can endure the difficulties of virus evolution, drug resistance, and zoonotic transmission by using synergistic interactions among plant components.

Moreover, the prospective influence of plant-based antivirals on worldwide health encompasses their function in fortifying immune responses and fostering general welfare. Plant-based chemicals have antiviral actions, but they also have immunomodulatory, anti-inflammatory, and antioxidant qualities that improve host defensive mechanisms against viral infections and boost immunological function. The body's natural defenses can be strengthened, resilience against viral threats can be improved, and holistic health and well-being can be promoted by including immune-boosting foods, herbal medicines, and lifestyle habits into daily routines. People can reduce their chance of catching viral illnesses and aid in the efforts of the international health community by adopting a preventative approach to health and wellness that places a high priority on dietary changes, lifestyle adjustments, and environmental variables. In summary, plant-based antivirals have the potential to have a substantial and wide-ranging influence on global health, providing comprehensive treatments to combat viral threats, foster resilience, and improve health equity globally. Researchers, legislators, medical professionals, and community stakeholders may lead the way in developing novel strategies for viral prevention, management, and treatment that are affordable, accessible, and culturally appropriate by utilizing the medicinal potential of plants. To fully realize the potential of plant-based antivirals as nature's response to viral threats, it is imperative to embrace nature's pharmacy, promote interdisciplinary collaborations, and prioritize health justice and environmental sustainability. Plant-based antivirals have the potential to change the course of global health, influence medical practice in the future, and build a more robust and healthy planet for future generations as research into them advances.

CHAPTER XIII

The Science of Viral Infections

Overview of common viral infections

With millions of victims globally and a high cost of morbidity and mortality, viral diseases present severe threats to global health. Viruses may spread quickly, cause widespread sickness, and put a strain on healthcare systems. This is true for everything from the common cold to more severe conditions like influenza, hepatitis, HIV/AIDS, and newly developing viral outbreaks like SARS-CoV-2. To effectively create therapies and harness nature's response to viral threats, one must have a thorough understanding of the epidemiology, clinical symptoms, transmission routes, and prevention measures of prevalent viral illnesses.

One of the most prevalent viral infections in the world, respiratory infections can cause a variety of respiratory symptoms, including fever, sore throats, coughs, congestion in the nasal passages, and exhaustion. Adenoviruses, parainfluenza viruses, coronaviruses, rhinoviruses, influenza viruses, and respiratory syncytial virus (RSV) are examples of respiratory viruses. Influenza is a seasonal respiratory illness that occurs by the influenza viruses A, B, and C. It may have grave repercussions, especially for high-risk groups like the elderly, small children, expecting mothers, and people with existing medical issues. Frequent antigenic changes in influenza viruses make yearly vaccination efforts necessary to keep up with circulating strains and stop outbreaks. In infants, older adults, and people with impaired immune systems, respiratory syncytial virus (RSV) is frequently the cause of respiratory infections that frequently result in pneumonia and bronchiolitis.

Adenoviruses and parainfluenza viruses can also cause respiratory infections, which can vary in severity from mild cold-like symptoms to serious lower respiratory tract infections. Another prevalent group of viral infections that impact millions of individuals worldwide is the hepatitis virus, which can cause varied degrees of liver damage and inflammation. Among the hepatitis viruses are hepatitis A, B, C, D, and E; each has a distinct mode of transmission, clinical presentation, and public health consequences. The primary way that the hepatitis A virus spreads is through tainted food and water. Acute hepatitis is characterized by symptoms like exhaustion, nausea, jaundice, and stomach discomfort. Airborne pathogens, such as the hepatitis B and hepatitis C viruses, are spread by direct contact with contaminated blood or body fluids or through mucosal contact. Hepatitis B or C virus infection over a prolonged period of time can cause liver cirrhosis, liver failure, and hepatocellular cancer, which makes managing and preventing the disease extremely difficult. In comparison to hepatitis B alone, hepatitis D virus replication requires coinfection with hepatitis B virus, which results in more severe liver disease. The fecal-oral route is the means by which the hepatitis E virus is spread, and it can result in acute or chronic hepatitis, especially in areas where sanitation and hygiene standards are low.

An estimated 38 million people worldwide are estimated to be living with HIV/AIDS, making HIV infection a serious health concern. HIV can be spread through intercourse, contaminated blood products, mother-to-child transmission during pregnancy, and needle sharing among injecting drug users. HIV infection develops in phases. Acute infection is marked by flu-like symptoms. Chronic infection follows, and if treatment is not received, the virus eventually develops into acquired immunodeficiency syndrome (AIDS). If antiretroviral therapy (ART) is not used to manage AIDS, it can result in high morbidity and mortality due to its hallmarks of severe immunosuppression, opportunistic infections, and cancers. HIV/AIDS continues to be a severe public health concern despite advancements in prevention and treatment, especially in areas with high prevalence and restricted access to medical care.

Emerging viral outbreaks underscore the potential for emerging viral infections to pose global challenges to health security. One such outbreak is the ongoing COVID-19 pandemic, which is being caused by SARS-CoV-2, a virus that causes severe acute respiratory syndrome. The coronavirus family of RNA viruses is varied and can infect both humans and animals. A number of coronaviruses have been linked to mild respiratory infections in people, including the common cold. Nonetheless, a number of coronaviruses have been linked to severe respiratory syndromes with elevated morbidity and mortality, such as SARS-CoV, MERS-CoV, and SARS-CoV-2. Rapid surveillance, early identification, containment strategies, vaccine development, and public health interventions are critical in limiting the spread of new viral diseases and their adverse effects on national and international health systems and economies. The COVID-19 pandemic has brought these strategies to light.

Other common viral disorders include gastrointestinal viral infections like norovirus and rotavirus, which cause gastroenteritis with symptoms like diarrhea, vomiting, abdominal pain, and dehydration. These infections are in addition to respiratory and bloodborne viruses. The highly contagious norovirus is frequently linked to outbreaks in places like long-term care institutions, schools, hospitals, and cruise ships. Around the world, rotavirus is the primary cause of severe diarrhea in infants and early children. This condition has a substantial impact on morbidity and mortality, especially in low-resource settings where access to clean water, sanitary conditions, and healthcare services is limited. In many countries, rotavirus vaccination has significantly decreased rotavirus-related morbidity and mortality. This shows how critical vaccination is for preventing viral infections and enhancing the health of children.

In summary, widespread viral infections represent severe threats to global health, impacting millions of individuals globally and resulting in a diverse array of clinical presentations, ranging from minor respiratory ailments to severe systemic diseases. To lessen the influence of frequent viral illnesses on public health and support nature's response to viral dangers, it is crucial to comprehend the epidemiology, transmission dynamics, clinical manifestations, and preventative tactics of these infections. Through the utilization of interdisciplinary techniques, cutting-edge technologies, and cooperative endeavors, scholars, medical practitioners, legislators, and communities can formulate efficacious therapies, capitalize on the medicinal properties of nature, and enhance health results for individuals and populations across the globe.

Mechanisms of viral replication and spread

Viral propagation and replication are intricate mechanisms that viruses exploit to enslave host cells, copy their genetic material, and create new viral offspring. To effectively design antiviral methods and use nature's response to viral threats, it is imperative to comprehend the mechanisms that underlie the replication and spread of viruses. Intricate tactics have been developed by viruses to subvert host immune responses, take advantage of biological machinery, and spread across host organisms. This has resulted in a wide range of viral illnesses with different clinical presentations and modes of transmission.

Viral entry into host cells, which entails attachment to particular cellular receptors and entry through endocytosis or membrane fusion, is the initial stage of viral replication. Various viruses use different entrance methods and receptors based on their host cell preferences and tropism. For instance, enveloped viruses, like coronaviruses and influenza viruses, attach to receptors on the surface of host cells through viral surface glycoproteins, which makes it easier for the virus to fuse with cell membranes and release its genetic material into the cytoplasm of the host cell. Through receptor- mediated endocytosis, non-enveloped viruses like adenovirus and norovirus enter host cells. Once inside endosomes, they release their genetic material into the cytoplasm to replicate.

Viral proteins and nucleic acids required for viral assembly and replication are produced by the replication, transcription, and translation of viral genetic material once it has entered the host cell. Viral RNA-dependent RNA polymerase (RdRp) or reverse transcriptase enzymes, which catalyze the synthesis of complementary RNA strands or DNA intermediates, respectively, are the tools used by RNA viruses, including the influenza virus, HIV, and hepatitis C virus, to replicate their genomes. DNA viruses, including adenoviruses and herpesviruses, exploit the host cell's DNA polymerase enzymes to replicate their genomes. This process frequently results in the development of viral DNA replication complexes inside the host cell's nucleus. To guarantee effective viral replication and assembly, these replication activities are closely controlled and synchronized with transcription factors, signaling pathways, and host cell cycle checkpoints.

Viral proteins are essential for controlling the activities of host cells, avoiding immune monitoring, and accelerating the growth and replication of viruses. In order to promote viral replication, a number of viruses encode viral proteins that disrupt host cell signaling pathways, thwart antiviral immune responses, and alter host cell machinery. For instance, the influenza virus encodes proteins called neuraminidase (NA) and hemagglutinin (HA), which, in addition to facilitating viral entrance and release from host cells, also inhibit host immune responses to enable viral reproduction. In a similar manner, to maintain persistent infection and elude immune clearance, the human immunodeficiency virus (HIV) produces viral proteins, including Tat, Rev, and Nef, that alter host cell transcription, translation, and immune evasion processes.

The packaging of freshly synthesized viral components into virions and their escape from host cells to infect new target cells or hosts are known as viral assembly and egress, and they are essential phases in the viral replication cycle. Viral glycoproteins and their lipid bilayer envelope are acquired by enveloped viruses during their frequent budding from host cell membranes. Viruses that are not enveloped usually leave their hosts by lysis or exocytosis, releasing their freshly formed virions into the extracellular space where they can infect nearby cells or find new hosts. Certain viruses, including herpesviruses and retroviruses, create latent or persistent infections in host cells, from which they can develop chronic or recurring viral illnesses by periodically reactivating and releasing infectious virions.

Numerous pathways, such as respiratory droplets, fecal-oral transmission, sexual contact, bloodborne transmission, and vertical transmission from mother to child, are involved in the propagation of viruses within host species. Respiratory droplets created during coughing, sneezing, or talking are the main way that respiratory viruses, such as influenza, respiratory syncytial virus (RSV), and coronaviruses, are spread. This can result in respiratory tract infections and airborne transmission. Enteric viruses, which frequently contaminate food, drink, or surfaces and cause gastrointestinal diseases, are transmitted through fecal-oral transmission. Examples of these viruses are norovirus and rotavirus. Bloodborne viruses that can cause systemic infections and potentially fatal consequences like liver cirrhosis and hepatocellular cancer are transferred through percutaneous or mucosal exposure to contaminated blood or bodily fluids. These viruses include the hepatitis C virus (HCV) and the hepatitis B virus (HBV).

In summary, viruses use complex mechanisms for reproduction and spread to infect new hosts or target cells, replicate within those cells, and expand their infection. Researchers can create tailored antiviral techniques that interrupt viral replication cycles, impede viral propagation, and stop viral transmission by comprehending the molecular principles behind transcription, translation, assembly, and egress of viruses. In order to effectively produce antiviral medicines and vaccines, it is necessary to employ interdisciplinary techniques that incorporate an understanding of viral pathophysiology, host-virus interactions, immunology, molecular biology, and drug development. This will allow nature to respond to viral threats. New understandings of viral replication mechanisms gained from virology research will guide the creation of creative therapies to fight viral infections and safeguard world health.

Impact of viral outbreaks on global health

Global health is significantly and widely impacted by viral epidemics, which frequently result in widespread disease, mortality, economic disruption, and social unrest. Viral outbreaks throughout history, including the 1918 influenza pandemic, the HIV/AIDS epidemic, the 2003 SARS outbreak, the 2014–2016 Ebola epidemic in West Africa, and the current COVID-19 pandemic brought on by the new coronavirus SARS–CoV–2, have highlighted how susceptible human populations are to newly emerging infectious diseases and the critical need for efficient measures to lessen their effects on public health. Comprehending the complex effects of viral breakouts on worldwide health is crucial for formulating all-encompassing measures, utilizing the natural defense mechanism against viral hazards, and constructing robust healthcare infrastructures that can avert, identify, and address subsequent viral pandemics.

The burden of illness and mortality that viral epidemics place on impacted communities is one of the most prominent and direct effects that they have. From minor respiratory symptoms to catastrophic systemic illness, infections caused by viruses can cause a wide range of clinical manifestations, depending on the virus's virulence, mode of transmission, and host susceptibility factors. Respiratory viruses such as influenza, coronaviruses, and respiratory syncytial virus (RSV) can cause pneumonia, respiratory failure, and acute respiratory distress syndrome (ARDS). These infections are hazardous for vulnerable groups like the elderly, young children, pregnant women, and people with underlying medical conditions. Liver cirrhosis, hepatocellular carcinoma, and immune suppression can be caused by bloodborne viruses that cause chronic infections, such as HIV, hepatitis B virus, and hepatitis C virus. Especially in young children and vulnerable people, intestinal viruses like rotavirus and norovirus can result in severe dehydration, electrolyte abnormalities, and gastrointestinal problems. The burden of viral morbidity and mortality is increased by inadequate infrastructure, unequal access to healthcare, and restricted access to healthcare services, which widens the wealth gap and exacerbates health inequities.

Furthermore, viral outbreaks have a significant negative socioeconomic impact on the lives, businesses, and social cohesiveness of the afflicted nations and communities.

Viral epidemics have a number of financial repercussions, such as direct medical costs, lost productivity from illness and absenteeism, disruptions to markets and supply chains, decreases in travel and tourism, and macroeconomic instability. For instance, millions of people experience unemployment, poverty, and food insecurity globally as a result of the COVID-19 epidemic, which has also resulted in widespread business closures, job losses, and economic slump. Viral outbreaks can produce economic shocks that exacerbate pre-existing socioeconomic inequality and widen them, particularly for small enterprises, informal workers, and underprivileged populations. Moreover, viral epidemics have the potential to overburden hospitals and medical staff, put pressure on the healthcare system, and take funds away from vital services like chronic illness treatment, maternity and child health, and immunizations. Viral outbreaks have socioeconomic effects that transcend beyond health systems and affect education, governance, and social cohesion. These effects have long-term effects on social stability, economic growth, and the fight against poverty.

Furthermore, viral outbreaks can have profound psychological and emotional effects on people as well as communities, leading to social isolation, shame, worry, and terror. Uncertainty about the spread of viruses, the severity of diseases, and containment strategies can increase stress and jeopardize mental health and well-being. In addition to making it more difficult to control the spread of viruses and ensure that everyone has equal access to healthcare services, stigmatization of afflicted people, communities, and healthcare professionals can worsen social exclusion, discrimination, and marginalization. Viral epidemics have long-term consequences on social cohesiveness, mental health, and resilience, in addition to their immediate adverse effects on health. This is especially true for vulnerable groups like frontline workers, refugees, migrants, and people with pre-existing mental health issues. Holistic strategies that put mental health care, community involvement, and social solidarity first are needed to address the psychosocial effects of viral outbreaks and promote social cohesion and resilience in the face of hardship.

Moreover, viral outbreaks underscore the necessity of coordinated worldwide responses to new infectious illnesses and the interdependence of global health security. Because viral infections are borderless and can spread quickly across continents through international travel and trade networks, global cooperation, information sharing, and coordinated action are crucial for pandemic planning and response. International organizations which include the World Health Assembly (or WHO for short the Agency for the Prevention and Control of Diseases, or CDC, and also other public health agencies, play a critical role in coordinating surveillance, monitoring, and response efforts to viral outbreaks in addition to offering affected countries technical assistance, capacity building, and resource mobilization.

The Global Health Security Agenda (GHSA), the Access to COVID-19 Tools (ACT) Accelerator, and the Coalition for Epidemic Preparedness Innovations (CEPI) are examples of multilateral initiatives that seek to improve pandemic preparedness, strengthen global health systems, and provide equitable access to viral disease vaccines, diagnostics, and treatments. By encouraging collaboration, solidarity, and shared responsibility, the international community can effectively counteract infectious threats, reduce their impact on global health, and build a more resilient and equitable society for coming generations.

In summary, viral epidemics pose complicated difficulties that necessitate comprehensive solutions and community action. They have far-reaching effects on global health, economy, and civilizations. By taking inspiration from nature's response to viral threats, policymakers, healthcare professionals, and the international community can develop effective strategies to prevent, detect, and respond to emerging infectious diseases by understanding the complex effects of viral outbreaks on health systems, economies, and communities. In an interconnected world, reducing the effect of viral outbreaks and enhancing global health security requires developing resilient healthcare systems, bolstering pandemic preparedness, and fostering health equity and social solidarity. In order to overcome the difficulties posed by viral outbreaks and create a better, more resilient society for all, it will be essential to promote cooperation, creativity, and solidarity as the globe works to contain the COVID-19 pandemic and gets ready for future viral threats.

CONCLUSION

Within the pages of "Nature's Answer to Viral Threats: Understanding the Potency of Plant-Based," the writers have carefully combed through the complex realm of plant-based treatments, revealing their immense potential in the fight against viral dangers. This book sheds light on the connections between contemporary medicine and the abundance of nature by combining scientific research with conventional wisdom. It presents a fascinating story of hope and fortitude in the face of viral pandemics by exploring diverse plant components' molecular mechanics and medicinal qualities.

This book's holistic approach pushes for a deeper comprehension of the symbiotic link between humans and the plant world beyond simple symptom relief. It emphasizes the importance of respecting nature's delicate balance and embracing its pharmacopeia. Furthermore, the insights offered to advocate for a more integrated and long-term approach to viral mitigation techniques, opening the door for a paradigm shift in healthcare.

Readers are left with a deep respect for the complex web of life and its endless potential to protect our health and well-being as the book's closing pages approach. In addition to being an academic discussion, "Nature's Answer to Viral Threats" is a ray of hope that encourages people and groups to use nature's medicine cabinet to combat viral enemies.

Thank you for buying and reading/ listening to our book. If you found this book useful/ helpful please take a few minutes and leave a review on the platform where you purchased our book. Your feedback matters greatly to us.

www.ingramcontent.com/pod-product-compliance
Lightning Source LLC
Chambersburg PA
CBHW050535160726
48003CB00002B/609